77313

£6.99

Carers Handbo

Caring for someone with diabetes

Marina Lewycka

AGE Concern

BOOKS

© 1999 Marina Lewycka
Published by Age Concern England
1268 London Road
London SW16 4ER

First published 1999

Editor   Marion Peat
Production   Vinnette Marshall
Designed and typeset by GreenGate Publishing Services, Tonbridge, Kent
Printed in Great Britain by Bell & Bain Ltd, Glasgow

A catalogue record for this book is available from the British Library.

ISBN 0-86242-282-5

Bulk orders

Age Concern England is pleased to offer customised editions of all its titles to UK companies, institutions or other organisations wishing to make a bulk purchase. For further information, please contact the Publishing Department at the address on this page. Tel: 0181-765 7200. Fax: 0181-765 7211. E-mail: addisom@ace.org.uk.

Contents

About the author

Marina Lewycka is a lecturer and freelance writer. She contributed to the BBC handbook *Who Cares Now?* and her training resource pack *Survival Skills for Carers* is published by the National Extension College with support from the Department of Health. She has been involved in the organisation of weekend courses for carers. She is also the author of three other books in the Carers Handbook Series.

Acknowledgements

I would like to thank the many people who have contributed to making this book. First of all, the people with diabetes and their carers, who have so generously shared their insights and experiences: Clive and Audrey, Jamil, Samina, Annie, Hazel, Val and Keith, Marie and Joe, Eleanor, Ron and Mary. Their words have helped add a human dimension to the dry facts, and their wisdom and honesty will give many others the inspiration to make the most of living with diabetes. I have changed some of their names to protect their confidentiality.

I would like to thank Lesley Hallett at the British Diabetic Association for her painstaking help in preparing the manuscript, and all the people at the BDA who gave such detailed and helpful advice on the content and wording, especially Norma McGough and Charlotte Hawkins.

Carolyn Taylor at the Sheffield Diabetes Centre spent hours going through my first draft, correcting my mistakes and sharing her experience of practical diabetes care, and Monica Sutton gave me invaluable advice about foot care.

Finally, I would like to thank the staff at Age Concern: Richard Holloway for his encouragement and support, Jeremy Fennell for his careful reading of the text, and Vinnette Marshall and Marion Peat for their help in completing the project.

Introduction

Diabetes is much more common than most people realise. It affects at least 1.4 million people in the UK, that's three out of every hundred adults. In fact the real number of people with diabetes could be even greater. According to the British Diabetic Association, for every person diagnosed with diabetes, there is another person with diabetes who is undiagnosed. Yet most of us, unless we know somebody with diabetes, are often unaware just how widespread it is.

If someone close to you develops diabetes, you suddenly realise just how much there is to learn about this mysterious and puzzling condition. Diabetes has been recognised since ancient times. It was recorded in ancient Egyptian hieroglyphics dating from about 1500 BC, and the difference between two types of diabetes was noted by doctors in India some 500 years ago. Attitudes to diabetes have changed over the years, and so have our understanding and the treatments available.

People often think of diabetes as a condition that affects young people and involves insulin injections. In fact, the great majority of people with diabetes are over 65, and have a type of diabetes that comes on gradually later in life. They may give themselves insulin injections, but they may be able to control their diabetes just with diet, or with a combination of diet and tablets. Some may have other health problems as well, or may develop complications as a result of their diabetes.

This book sets out to bring you up-to-date information about diabetes and ways of controlling it. It is aimed at people close to or caring for someone with diabetes, maybe their partner, or an elderly parent or relative. It draws on the experiences of people with diabetes and their carers to tell you what you can expect, and what the person you care for may be feeling and experiencing. And it gives practical information and advice about managing diabetes. For, as Audrey says (p 1), 'Diabetes is something you have to live with, but it's not something that has to take over your life.'

1 Understanding diabetes

Diabetes is a very common condition, which affects about one in fifty people in Britain, most of them in their 60s and 70s. It happens when there is too much glucose (a form of sugar) in the blood. This may be because the body is not producing enough of the hormone that controls blood sugar, called insulin, or because the insulin it produces is not working properly.

Fortunately we now understand much more about how to control and treat diabetes, so although it is still a serious condition, most people with diabetes can continue to live full and active lives. This chapter explains why diabetes happens and how different types of diabetes affect people.

Audrey

'I was diagnosed with diabetes ten years ago when I was 62. I knew something was wrong, I felt so tired and ill, and I was losing weight. In a way it came as a relief to know what it was. Diabetes doesn't stop me from doing anything I want to do. Yes, I do have to eat a healthy diet, but that's something I would choose to do anyway.

'I would say to anyone who is told they have diabetes – don't panic. It's not the end of the world. Diabetes is something you have to live with, but it's not something that has to take over your life.'

Coming to terms with the diagnosis

If you have a friend or a relative who has just been diagnosed with diabetes, you may be wondering what you can do to help. As Audrey says, the first thing is not to panic.

Finding out you have diabetes can be very distressing, and can make people withdrawn and depressed for a while. Some people describe the time after they first learn they have diabetes as a period of grieving, rather like bereavement. If you are living with or caring for someone who has recently been told they have diabetes, you can help them to understand that this grieving is natural. You can explain that it is not a sign of weakness, and the mood will gradually lift as they learn to manage their condition and start to feel better.

Jamil

'My grandfather and my father and my brother all have diabetes, so at one level I always knew I would be more likely to get it. But it still came as a terrible shock. I suppose you always hope you'll be the one who doesn't get it. I felt so depressed. I just kept thinking about all the things I wouldn't be able to do from now on.'

Sometimes the carer is aware something is wrong long before the person with diabetes will admit it.

Annie

Annie knew there was something wrong with Ernest, because he was always very thirsty, and seemed drowsy most of the time. But she had to plead with him to go to the doctor.

'He was very stubborn. He said, "There's nothing wrong with me." In the end I pleaded with him, so he said "Oh, all right. Just for you." When he came back he seemed very gloomy. "How did you get on?" I asked. "Oh," he said, "It's all a lot of rubbish. He said I've got to come back on Thursday, and bring my wife. He thinks I've got diabetes." "Well, I'm not surprised," I said, "You've always had a fancy for anything sweet." "I know," he said. "That's why I picked you."'

(Most people, like Annie and Ernest, used to believe there was a link between diabetes and eating sweet things. In fact this is one of the major myths about diabetes.)

For the carer, too, finding out that someone close to them has diabetes can be distressing. It may mean a change of plans, difficult decisions to be faced, even relationships to be reassessed.

Marie

Marie was 62 years old when she discovered her husband Joe had diabetes. He was already quite severely ill when it was diagnosed.

'I woke up one morning, and Joe wasn't there. I had no idea what had happened to him. In fact he'd got up early and gone to the doctor's surgery. His toes had gone black, and that really frightened him, but he didn't say anything to me. The next I saw of him, he was in hospital.'

Marie's husband had to have three toes amputated. He also has trouble with his eyesight and is having laser treatment. Marie finds she has become a full-time carer.

'We didn't have an easy marriage. He was always saying, when I retire, we're going to do this, or we're going to do that. I was looking forward to travelling, seeing the world. Instead, I'm looking after an invalid. It makes me quite bitter.'

Many problems with diabetes arise because it is diagnosed too late, and damage has already been done. But although diabetes cannot be cured, it can be very successfully controlled. There is help, support and advice available from health professionals and through social services. However, the key people who can do most to manage the condition and keep complications at bay are the person with diabetes and their carer.

Understanding diabetes

This section will help you understand more about what happens in the body when someone has diabetes.

Our bodies need a steady amount of glucose (a form of sugar) to give us energy. When we eat starchy or sugary foods they are broken down into glucose and enter the bloodstream. A hormone called *insulin*, which is made in the pancreas, helps the body's cells to take up the glucose from the blood and turn it into energy. The insulin is an 'enabling' hormone – it is a bit like a key that unlocks the door of the cell and lets the glucose in.

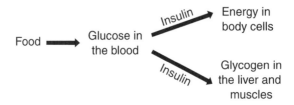

If there is more glucose than we require for our immediate energy needs, the surplus is stored in our liver and muscles. Insulin also helps to take the glucose out of the bloodstream and into the liver and muscles where it is stored as glycogen. When we need more energy, either because we have been exercising or because we have not eaten for a while, glucose is released from the liver and goes back into the bloodstream. Maintaining the right level of glucose in the blood is a delicately balanced cycle, in which the hormone insulin plays an essential part.

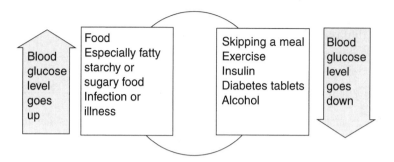

Some people cannot maintain this balance. When the balance breaks down, diabetes is the result. The balance can break down because the body is not producing enough insulin, or because the insulin is not working properly. If this happens, the glucose we get from our food does not go into the body cells or the liver. Instead the levels of glucose in our blood become very high and some of the glucose is passed out of the body in our urine when we go to the toilet. When we need more energy, because we have been exercising or because we have not eaten for a while, we cannot use the glucose in our liver. Instead, we may draw on the energy stored in our body fat, causing us to lose weight. But this is not enough, and we will begin to feel tired and weak.

Symptoms of diabetes

The most common symptom of diabetes is a general feeling of tiredness and weakness. This happens because the body cannot take glucose up into the cells and convert it into energy. Other symptoms include feeling very thirsty and passing urine a lot, as the body washes the high levels of glucose out of the blood into the urine. People with diabetes may also find themselves losing weight, and they may notice a tingling in their hands and feet, and blurred vision. Infections, skin problems, and itchiness in the genital area caused by fungal infections can also be signs of diabetes.

Because these symptoms seem very general, and tend to come on gradually in older people, they may not go to the doctor or get their diabetes diagnosed for quite a while.

Hazel

Hazel's mother had quite severe symptoms by the time she was diagnosed with diabetes. 'Mum was very thirsty all the time and drinking a lot, but we didn't think anything of it. We thought it was just because it was so warm in their flat. Then she started to get pins and needles in her feet, and she started to bang her feet all the time – they were always painful and always cold. This went on for a couple of years before the diabetes was diagnosed. When they told her, she said, "Oh, that's why my feet have been so funny."'

Different types of diabetes

There are two main types of diabetes that can affect people.

Type 1 diabetes, or Insulin Dependent Diabetes Mellitus (IDDM), is sometimes called 'juvenile onset diabetes', because it is usually diagnosed in younger people below the age of 30. It tends to come on suddenly as the cells that produce insulin in the pancreas stop working and no insulin at all is produced. People with type 1 diabetes are completely dependent on insulin injections. No-one knows exactly why the insulin-producing cells break down, but one theory is that it is triggered by a viral infection.

Type 2 diabetes, or Non-Insulin Dependent Diabetes Mellitus (NIDDM) tends to affect people as they get older. Three-quarters of those who are diagnosed with it are aged over 60, and for this reason it is sometimes called 'maturity onset diabetes'. It shows itself gradually, as the pancreas produces less insulin, or the insulin that is produced works less effectively. Again, we do not know quite why this happens, but weight, diet, exercise and family history may all play a part. People with type 2 diabetes can often control their blood glucose level just by being very careful about what they eat and when, or by taking tablets as well as changing their diet. But about one in four people who have type 2 diabetes can control their blood glucose level better if they take insulin.

As well as these two common forms of diabetes, there are a number of other types of diabetes which are very rare in this country, but which you may hear spoken about. These include diabetes brought on by malnutrition, and *diabetes insipidus*, a disorder of the pituitary gland that causes excessive urination. This is quite distinct from diabetes mellitus, as blood glucose level is not involved.

Diabetes and older people

Diabetes is more common in older people, and the older someone gets, the more they are at risk. It is hard to put a figure on exactly how many people are affected, because many who have diabetes do not realise it. Scientists estimate that for every person diagnosed with diabetes there could be another one who has it but does not know it. At least six people out of every hundred aged over 65 have diabetes – and of these, between 75 per cent and 90 per cent will have type 2 diabetes.

Asian people and Afro-Caribbean people are particularly at risk from middle age onwards, though it is not clear why. Diet and genetic links are both being studied as possible reasons.

People who have had diabetes for a while before they are actually diagnosed, and people who have had type 1 diabetes for many years are more at risk of developing complications. This is why it is especially important for people with diabetes to keep healthy with a routine of diet, exercise and careful monitoring of blood glucose level.

For more *i*nformation

ℹ Call the British Diabetic Association Careline on 0171-636 6112.

ℹ *Balance for Beginners* (two versions are available, depending on whether diabetes is type 1 or type 2 – specify which you would like), published by the British Diabetic Association

ℹ *Living with Diabetes for those Treated with Insulin* and *Living with Diabetes for those Treated with Diet and Tablets*, by Dr John Day, published on behalf of the British Diabetic Association by John Wiley & Son.

2 Day-to-day diabetes care

Caring for someone with diabetes is a team effort. This chapter looks at some of the professionals who will be looking after your relative, and at your own role as a carer. But the most important member of the diabetes care team is the person with diabetes. Research shows that by carefully monitoring and controlling their blood glucose level, they can help keep the damaging complications of diabetes to a minimum. This chapter also looks at how blood glucose monitoring is done, and how you can help.

Mary

'Ron has diabetes and I have difficulty walking as a result of a hip operation. So we care for each other, really. I check his feet every day, because he can't see very well. He does all the vacuuming, and he takes me out in the car. He puts the washing out if it's a nice day. I cook his meals. When you're together all the time, it's easy to get irritable. But we do have separate interests.'

Living with diabetes

No two people with diabetes are alike. Some people find that their blood glucose level settles down almost at once when treatment begins, while others find it swings wildly between very high and so low that they are in danger of having a 'hypo' (there is more about 'hypos' in Chapter 8, pp 89–96). When diabetes is first diagnosed, the doctor will probably spend some time working out the best programme of treatment for the individual, with the aim of bringing their blood glucose level down and keeping it stable.

There are three main treatments that can help someone with diabetes to get the blood glucose balance right:

1 **Diet** Eating regular meals containing starchy carbohydrate foods such as bread and potatoes helps to control blood glucose levels. Some people can control their blood glucose level just through their diet, but diet is equally important for people who are also taking tablets or insulin. There is more about eating a healthy diet in Chapter 3.

2 **Tablets** Some people can take tablets to lower the level of glucose in the blood. There is more about tablets and how they work in Chapter 4.

3 **Insulin injections** These replace insulin that the body can no longer produce. There are many different types of insulin. These are described in Chapter 5.

The doctor can refer someone with diabetes to a state registered dietitian for advice on a diet, or prescribe tablets with the diet, or may put the person straight onto insulin. The treatments prescribed will be based on the individual's circumstances.

The doctor or diabetes specialist nurse will also advise the person or their carer about monitoring the blood glucose level regularly. If it seems to be going too high or too low on a regular basis, contact the doctor or the diabetes specialist nurse.

What to expect from the Health Service

Some people are treated for diabetes at their GP's surgery. Others attend a clinic at a hospital or at a health centre. This will depend on what local resources are available for people with diabetes.

There are advantages to both. Some GPs have a good knowledge of diabetes and are expert at treating it; they also know the patient and their family, and the GP's surgery may be more convenient. On the other hand, if the GP is not a specialist in diabetes care, the special diabetes clinic may provide a better service. Some people attend both a clinic at the hospital and also see their GP regularly.

Annie

'Our GP has a special interest in diabetes and runs a clinic, so we go there every week. Once a year, we see the doctor, but most of the time it's the specialist nurse who looks after us. She's very knowledgeable, and she's become like a friend. I can ring her up about anything. But we also go up to see the consultant at the hospital once a year, and the nurse from the hospital clinic visits us regularly. They all seem to work together.'

The quality of the care will vary from area to area, and from practice to practice.

Eleanor

'I don't feel the GP has time for me. When I first started to have problems with my eyes, I was worried about losing my sight. I went to see him because I noticed a bit of bleeding in my eye. He said, "Oh that's nothing, it's just a little blood vessel." He made me feel as though I was wasting his time. But there's another doctor there in the practice who specialises in diabetes, and he's much more helpful. I always try and make an appointment to see him now.'

Most GPs provide the same level of care as you would get in hospital. But if you are not satisfied with the care your GP gives, you could try to see another doctor in the practice, or move to another practice. To do this, you simply have to register with another practice. They will then write to your former GP to get your notes. You do not have to give any reasons unless you want to. You can get a list of local GPs from the Health Authority or from your local Community Health Council (called Health Councils in Scotland), or ask at your local library.

When diabetes is first diagnosed

When someone is first diagnosed with diabetes, they should also get a full medical check-up. This will show whether they have any other medical problems as well as their diabetes. (These may be linked to diabetes, or they may be completely separate.) The medical check-up should include:

- measurement of weight and height;
- urine test;
- blood test and blood glucose measure (as basis for long-term control);
- blood pressure check;
- eye examination;
- foot examination.

Diabetes is a complex illness, and there are many things someone newly diagnosed with diabetes needs to know. After they have been diagnosed, everyone with diabetes should get advice from a nurse or doctor, and education about:

- what diabetes is, and how the treatment will help to control it;
- any changes to their diet, on the advice of a state registered dietitian;
- exercise, stopping smoking, and controlling their weight;
- how diabetes could affect other aspects of their life, for example their job, relationships and family, driving, insurance, prescription charges, etc;
- where to get help and support, including local support groups and the British Diabetic Association.

If someone is being treated with insulin, they will be shown the best way to inject themselves. If they are being treated with tablets, they will be told about how and when to take them.

People treated with insulin and/or tablets will also be told about what happens if their blood glucose level goes too low and they have a 'hypo'. There is more about how to recognise a 'hypo' in Chapter 8.

Regular check-ups

People with diabetes should have an annual check-up at the clinic or surgery. But you can contact the doctor, practice nurse or diabetes specialist nurse whenever there is a problem, for example if symptoms seem to be getting worse, or the blood glucose level stays high, or the person is getting a lot of 'hypos'.

Everyone with diabetes should have an eye examination every year. Eye tests at the opticians are free for people with diabetes, but they will have to pay for lenses for their glasses. The annual eye examination is not the same as the visit to the optician – it is to check for signs of retinopathy (an eye condition which is discussed on p 73).

Some complications of diabetes do not have many symptoms in the early stages. It is easy to feel so much better after treatment has started that some people do not to bother with follow-up check-ups. If you are caring for someone with diabetes, you can help by making sure they see the nurse or doctor for regular check-ups. They should also have an annual eye examination and see the chiropodist regularly so that any problems can be identified and dealt with straightaway.

Other professionals who can help

As well as the doctor at the clinic and your GP, you will come across quite a number of different professionals in the course of your relative's illness. These include:

Hospital consultant Patients who have particular problems or complications may be referred by their GP to a consultant at the hospital. Sometimes they will see a diabetes specialist, but they may also see an ophthalmologist (eye specialist), nephrologist (kidney specialist), cardiologist (heart specialist), neurologist (specialist in disorders of the nervous system) or surgeon, depending on their problems.

Diabetes specialist nurse The nurse at the diabetes clinic will be very knowledgeable about diabetes, and will be able to give you excellent advice about all aspects of diabetes control. She will also give information about taking tablets or injecting insulin, if necessary. She will be able to advise about the most suitable devices for monitoring blood glucose and injecting insulin, and how to cope with illness and make day-to-day adjustments in taking insulin. She will explain what a 'hypo' feels like and what to do when one starts to come on. The specialist nurse is the best person to ring for day-to-day advice.

State registered chiropodist She/he will check the feet, trim the toenails if necessary, and give advice about foot care and buying shoes. Someone with diabetes should check their feet every day and see a state registered chiropodist regularly, especially if they are unable to care for their feet or have a particular problem.

State registered dietitian When diabetes is first diagnosed, the person should always ask to see a dietitian. The dietitian won't just tell them what foods to eat and what to avoid, but will look at the foods they like to eat, and suggest ways that they could adapt them and fit them in to their new healthy eating programme. It's best if the partner or carer is there too, as changing someone's diet will affect the whole household. If you have any particular problems or questions about diet, the dietitian will be able to give you expert advice.

Ophthalmologist Regular eye examinations can detect the complications of diabetes that can lead to loss of sight if left untreated. Most people with diabetes should have their eyes examined when they are first diagnosed, and then have them regularly checked each year. But if someone has eye problems they will need to see the ophthalmologist more often.

Social worker Sometimes a person with diabetes has problems about where they live or whether they can manage at home. A social worker can advise them about what help they are entitled to at home, and can also help them decide whether they should go into a residential or nursing home. There is more about this in Chapter 9.

However, the most important members of the diabetes care team are the person with diabetes, and the person who cares for them. Keeping up the routine of urine or blood glucose monitoring, healthy eating and medication can sometimes seem like hard work – and everyone has lapses from time to time – but it's worth making the effort to avoid some of the complications that can arise if diabetes is not properly controlled.

Minimising the risk of complications

Before insulin was discovered in 1922, most people who had diabetes did not live very long, so little was understood about the complications that could arise from diabetes over a period of time.

Nowadays some people live with diabetes for more than 50 years without any complications. But there is more risk of developing complications the longer someone has diabetes.

There may be damage to small blood vessels, affecting the eyes, the nerves and the kidneys. Or there may be damage to large blood vessels affecting the circulation, and leading to problems with legs and feet, and increasing the risk of heart disease and strokes. There is more about this in Chapter 6.

However, the good news is that the risk of complications can be greatly reduced if the person's weight, blood glucose levels and blood pressure are carefully controlled. This is where the person with diabetes and their carer have such an important part to play.

Unfortunately some people find out too late that they have diabetes, so the damage has already been done. In some cases, complications such as retinopathy will have led to the diagnosis of diabetes. Even so, good treatment and careful control of blood glucose level and blood pressure can stop things getting worse.

Getting the blood glucose level right

The key to controlling diabetes is to get just the right balance between the amount of glucose in the blood, and the amount of insulin needed to take the glucose out of the blood and into the cells of the body, where it is used for energy. Too much glucose in the blood and someone with diabetes will experience tiredness, dizziness, thirst, passing a lot of urine – all the symptoms of hyperglycaemia. Too little glucose and they may feel faint or dizzy or have a 'hypo'. (There is more about this in Chapter 8.)

■ Things that *raise* the blood glucose level are eating (especially sugary and starchy foods); infection and illness; some prescribed drugs.

■ Things that *lower* the blood glucose level are: skipping a meal, exercise, alcohol, insulin and certain tablets (more information about tablets is given in Chapter 4).

In people who do not have diabetes, the body works out the right balance minute by minute by regulating the amount of insulin released from the pancreas. In people with diabetes, this automatic balancing act no longer happens. Instead the doctor or specialist nurse has to work out the exact amount of insulin or tablets someone needs to take to balance the amount and type of food they eat. This is more difficult because people's eating and exercise patterns are bound to vary every day and at different times of day. Regular monitoring can help someone see whether they have got the right balance.

Monitoring blood glucose level at home

Most people without diabetes have a blood glucose level between 4 and 8 mmol/l (this is a technical term meaning millimols per litre). However, do not feel downhearted if the person you care for goes above this level. So long as they keep their blood glucose level down below 10 or 11 most of the time, there is no need to worry. The doctor or nurse will tell the person you care for what is a realistic target. However, if the reading is regularly higher than this it is best to talk to the nurse about how it can be better controlled.

You can monitor diabetes control by urine testing and blood glucose testing. Most people with diabetes regularly test their own blood glucose level at home by pricking their finger and testing the blood on a special strip. It is also possible to buy electronic machines that give an automatic reading. Ask the nurse which is the best machine for you to use.

Mary

'I always make sure Ron does his blood sugar test before he goes to bed at night. He has a little instrument called a Glucotrend Soft-test, and he says he hardly feels it.'

How to test

There are now so many devices on the market to make finger-pricking easier and less painful that you are spoilt for choice. Lancets are available on prescription, but the more hi-tech gadgets you will need to buy for yourself. You can find out more about the range of finger-pricking gadgets from the specialist nurse or from your pharmacist, or you can send off for them by post. Talk to your diabetes specialist nurse or GP before you buy one. The British Diabetic Association also has information about the range of products available, and their magazine *Balance* has details of suppliers. Some clinics will let you borrow a monitor to try out before you buy it.

Read the instructions that come with the device carefully, as they are all different. If you are caring for someone who is monitoring their own blood glucose level, it is very important that you follow the manufacturers' instructions, and that the person doing the monitoring has been trained by their health care professionals. It is surprising how many people make mistakes in reading their blood glucose level.

Hazel

'I do my Mum's blood glucose monitoring for her – she doesn't like doing it herself. The diabetes specialist nurse got me a little machine so I wouldn't have to stab – she said it would be better for Mum. I've been doing it three times a day, just after breakfast, before lunch and after lunch. They've got it down to 17 and it's gradually coming down. But she keeps getting chest infections and urinary infections, and that puts it up again.'

How often?

When someone is first diagnosed with diabetes, they may need to test their blood several times a day. As a pattern emerges, and the blood glucose level is stabilised, they may be able to test less regularly. Some people only test their blood glucose level once a week. But if there are any changes in the person's circumstances – such as illness or a change of activities or a change of diet or medication – the blood glucose level may go up or down quite sharply, so it will be necessary to test more often. The specialist nurse will advise you about how often to test.

What about urine tests?

Some people prefer to check their diabetes control by testing their urine. This is done by dipping a special strip into urine, and watching how it changes colour. Some people can get an accurate reading from testing their urine, but on the whole the finger-pricking method is much more accurate. This is because the level at which glucose spills out into the urine varies from person to person. The relationship between blood and urine concentrations is not very precise. The diabetes care team can advise on the best way for someone to monitor their diabetes control.

Getting the right balance

Keeping the right blood glucose level can prevent long-term damage and complications of diabetes. It usually makes the person with diabetes feel much healthier and livelier. However, if the blood glucose level dips too low the result may be a 'hypo' (see pp 89–96).

It isn't easy to get the blood glucose balance exactly right. Most people with diabetes either err on the high side, with a slightly increased risk of complications and long-term damage from diabetes, or they can err on the low side, and risk having 'hypos' more often. Quality of life is a very individual thing, and in the end it is up to each person to discuss with their diabetes care team and settle on a balance which they can most happily live with.

Is it available on prescription?

People with diabetes can get free prescriptions if they are being treated with insulin or tablets, but not if they are being treated with diet alone.

Available on prescription:

- Insulin (including cartridges).
- Tablets.
- Syringes and needles.
- Lancets for finger-pricking.
- Testing strips.

Not available on prescription:

- Blood glucose level monitoring meters.
- Finger-pricking devices.
- Pen needles.

Pens themselves are usually available free from the manufacturers, and are supplied through the clinic.

Pen needles will hopefully be available on prescription by the time this book is published. Check their availability with your diabetes care team.

Don't forget to care for the carer (that's you!)

With all the attention focused on the person with diabetes, the carer can sometimes feel like a spare part. Caring is a difficult and stressful job, yet carers often feel that their efforts are not recognised.

Marie

Marie found being a carer was taking over her whole life. 'It's a very undermining thing to be a carer. You're a second class citizen. When we go out with him in his wheelchair people always ask, how is he? How's he getting on? They never ask about me. It's as if I don't exist except to care for him. And yet my own health has suffered as a result. I've got asthma and angina because of the stress.'

Some people become carers gradually, as their spouse or parent becomes more ill and dependent. Other people find a sudden event or crisis turns their life upside down and plunges them into a caring role, which they did not expect and may resent. If your relationship with the person you care for was difficult, you are more likely to have negative feelings about caring for them.

Marie

'People think caring for someone is just doing a bit of cooking or cleaning, but it's more than that. He can't walk by himself, so I have to take him out in his trolley. He can't even balance to wash himself, so I have to wash him down below.

'I used to have a little job, but I had to give that up. I came back home and he was standing in the doorway crying. He'd fallen down the stairs. Now we don't go out much at all. I feel the four walls closing in on me. We live from meal to meal. There's nothing but meals and television. If it's fine we go out for a walk in the park. But most of the time he just sits there as if he's waiting to die. It's wearing me down.'

Not everyone's experiences are as bleak as Marie's, but most people have times when they feel very low. How you feel about caring for someone with diabetes will depend on your relationship with the person, and on how much care they need. You may be caring for an older parent or relative, or for a spouse with whom you've shared the ups and downs of married life. But almost everybody who ends up caring for someone else has times when they feel they can't cope.

Hazel

Hazel looks after her mother who is 80 years old and has had diabetes for six years, and also for her father who is 85, and has health problems. 'I'm caring for both of them. I pop in most days – I had to give up my job to do the caring. If I was at work I couldn't just drop everything and go when she needs me.

'I feel I should be there all the time, but I've my own family to see to. Of late I feel as if I'm not handling it well – I feel as if she's draining all my energy out of me. But she always feels better when I've been.

'Once I took them away with us on holiday. We rented a chalet for a week. But there were three lots of beds to make, as well as all the cooking and clearing up. By the end of the week I was shattered.'

Getting a break

Sometimes the carer and the person they care for need a break from each other.

Val and Keith

Val has had diabetes since she was a teenager, and now in her late 50s, she has had both legs amputated and has kidney dialysis four times a day. Her husband Keith cares for her, but even with her disabilities Val cherishes her independence.

'When Val first came home from hospital after she'd had her legs amputated, I wouldn't go anywhere', says Keith. 'I wouldn't leave her for ten minutes. I was completely over the top. I thought I had to be there all the time in case something happened.

'But now I realise it's important to have a break. And Val needs a break too. She doesn't need me fussing over her all the time, and it's amazing what she can do – with the proper equipment she can dress and bath herself. We went out for a meal recently with some friends, and Val went off to the disabled toilet by herself. Our friend came running after her, but I said, "It's all right, she can manage on her own."'

Val says, 'But when I'm really poorly I need looking after. And then he's there, at my beck and call all the time, doing my meals, my dialysis, my injections.'

If you really feel you can't leave the person you care for, there are 'sitting services' in many areas, where someone will come in and sit with the person you care for while you go out for a couple of hours. You can find out about sitting services through your local authority's social services department.

Respite care

When caring is getting too much for you and you need a break of more than a couple of hours, respite care could be the answer. Respite care could mean day care, when the person you care for goes to a day centre during the day and comes back home in the evening. This could be once or twice a week, or it could be every day. At the day centre, there will be activities and opportunities to meet other people, meals will be provided and there may be facilities for personal care such as bathing.

Annie

Annie could cope with her husband's diabetes, but when he started to develop Alzheimer's disease as well, she found that looking after him at home all day was more than she could manage.

'He used to go wandering off all the time, and I was having to run down the road to fetch him back. But I have a heart condition. In the end, I was having to lock him in. It was heartbreaking. Social services arranged for him to go into day care at a lady's house once a week. Then he started going two days a week to another centre. In the end he was going every day. It was lonely on my own, but I could cope better. Then they suggested he could go into respite care for a week every month. But I said, No. I fought them all the way. But it got that bad, he was weeing on the floor, and sometimes he would get violent. I had to let him go in the end.'

Another form of respite care is when the person you care for goes away to a residential or nursing home for a week or two. This can be ideal if you need to go away on holiday – it can be a holiday for them too. But older people can resent residential respite care, as they sometimes see it as the first step towards permanent full-time residential care. So if you suggest it, you may meet with some resistance.

Hazel

'I got my Mum into respite care. It was a lovely home in a country village not far from here. She was in tears when they took her in, though they bent over backwards to be nice to her. But she was very naughty. She had her own room, and she just sat in it, feeling sorry for herself. She wouldn't mix with anybody, and when I came to see her she wouldn't talk to me, she just ignored me. She was only there for a week – she refused to go for a fortnight – and when she came back she said she'd never go again.

I thought I'd be able to have a nice rest, but it was nothing but worry all week.'

You can find out about respite care from your local authority's social services department, and you may get some help towards the cost. Or you could arrange it privately through a residential or nursing home that you know.

Survival guide for carers

If you are caring for someone, don't forget that you also have to care for yourself.

- ▓ Make sure you have time to yourself during the day. Develop outside friends and interests.
- ▓ Find out if there is a carers' support group in your area – contact the British Diabetic Association or the Carers National Association (addresses on pp 124 and 125).
- ▓ If you feel very stressed or pressured, talk to your GP.
- ▓ Contact the social services department for an assessment of your relative's needs. They may be able to arrange help at home or respite care. (There is more about this in Chapter 9.)
- ▓ Under the Carers' Act (1995) you are entitled to an assessment of your own needs when the person you care for is assessed. If you feel you are not coping, contact your local social services department and ask for help – you are entitled to it by right.
- ▓ Make sure the person you care for is claiming all the allowances and benefits they are entitled to. Attendance Allowance is one of the most under-claimed benefits. Some people under 65 may be able to claim Incapacity Benefit or Disability Living Allowance. You may be entitled to Invalid Care Allowance if you are of working age and are caring for someone for more than 35 hours a week. The Citizens Advice Bureau, or the social worker or your local Benefits Agency (DSS) office can advise you.

How the British Diabetic Association (BDA) can help

One of the worst things about finding out you have diabetes is suddenly feeling that you are different to everybody around you. Someone who has just been diagnosed with diabetes may feel upset, angry, frightened and alone. They may have lots of questions they want to ask, but feel too embarrassed to ask the doctor or nurse. The carer, too, may be worried about the long-term implications of this condition, and how it will affect the whole family. This is where the BDA comes in.

Through its network of local groups, it can put people with diabetes and their carers in touch with each other. Some groups arrange regular meetings and talks, others give each other support by telephone. They may swap hints about treatment and monitoring, or pass on recipes, or just get together for a good talk.

The BDA also provides a confidential **Careline** service, which takes general enquiries from people with diabetes, their carers and health care professionals. You can contact the Careline by phone on 0171-636 6112 (9am to 5pm, Monday to Friday), or write to them care of the BDA at the address below, or e-mail them on careline@diabetes.org.uk.

Nationally, the BDA publishes up-to-date advice about living with diabetes and keeps you informed about the latest research. It also supports and funds several research projects.

To find out about your nearest BDA group, ask at the clinic or contact them directly at British Diabetic Association, 10 Queen Anne Street, London W1M 0BD. Tel: 0171-323 1531. Fax: 0171-637 3644.

Keith

'We've been in the BDA for quite a few years now. We get the BDA magazine, and it's always got loads of information, and new menus and recipes to try. I like reading about other people's experiences. You get leaflets and free brochures, and you find out about events. But for us, the main thing has been the local BDA branch. When Val was the secretary, people sometimes used to ring us up for advice, and it was good to feel you could help others. We learn from each other's experiences. I think it's especially important if you've just been diagnosed – you want another person with diabetes to talk to. The branch also invites speakers in to come to our meetings and give a presentation on health, diet and general interest subjects, so making a good social event.'

For more *i*nformation

i The British Diabetic Association (BDA) produces a range of information leaflets, including *Diabetes Care Today*; *Diabetes and You: A guide for the older person*; *Diabetes Care: What you should expect*; *Diabetes: What care to expect in hospital* and *Diabetes, the BDA and You*.

3 Healthy eating, healthy living

Healthy eating is the key to diabetes control – even if someone is taking insulin or tablets as well. People diagnosed with diabetes often worry that they will have to completely change their eating habits, and to eat lots of different and special foods. In fact people with diabetes are advised to eat the same healthy diet that is recommended for everybody. But healthy eating is only a part of it. Being the right weight, getting enough exercise and giving up smoking are important too.

Audrey

'I wouldn't say that diabetes has stopped me eating anything I like. In fact it's introduced me to all kinds of new foods I didn't eat much before, such as pasta and rice. One of our favourites is pasta with home made sauce. It's delicious. We don't bother with the special diabetic foods at all. They're a waste of money.'

Choosing the right foods

Eating is one of the great pleasures of life, and just because someone has diabetes doesn't mean that has to change. But choosing foods that make up a healthy diet as well as being delicious is especially important for someone with diabetes.

The food we eat is converted into glucose that goes into our bloodstream to give our body energy. So the type and amount of food we eat affects both the level of glucose in our blood, and our weight – which are both important things to control.

People with diabetes should eat regular meals based on starchy foods like bread and potatoes. They should try to eat more fruit and vegetables, and cut down on fat. It is important to limit sugar, and cut out sugar in drinks, but it is not necessary to cut out sugar altogether. However, cutting down on sugary foods like cakes and biscuits is important if the person is overweight.

Annie

When Annie's husband was diagnosed with diabetes she didn't waste any time.

'He came home from the doctor and said, "Make us a cup of coffee, love." But I said, "No, you're not having any more of that coffee – not with four spoons of sugar in it." Then I went straight down to the chemist and got some of those artificial sweeteners. That was on the Monday. When we went back on the Thursday his blood glucose level had gone down from 22 to 11. The nurse said, "By gum, you've been quick!"'

How the dietitian can help

When someone is first diagnosed with diabetes, they should get an appointment to see a dietitian. If the carer helps with shopping or cooking, they should be involved too. The dietitian will look at the kinds of meals the person already eats and suggest ways of adapting them to make them healthier, or she/he will suggest alternatives that are just as tasty but much better for you.

Introducing change gradually

It isn't easy to change the eating habits of a lifetime overnight. Sometimes older people find it particularly hard to make the change to new foods. If you try too hard to make someone eat things they don't want, they will simply become stubborn or find ways of 'cheating'. It's much better to start with one or two simple changes like using artificial (intense) sweeteners instead of sugar in drinks and gradually introducing a healthier balance into their existing diet by including more fruit and vegetables or cutting down on butter and other full fat dairy foods. You can soon get used to a casserole with some beans added, and a little less meat. You don't have to have wholemeal bread all of the time – enjoy a variety of different breads. It is important to eat more fibre, but that doesn't mean having 'brown' everything.

Val

'When I was the secretary of the local British Diabetic Association, I found it was the older people who just couldn't give up their sweets and treats. I've had diabetes since I was eighteen, so I had years to get used to eating a healthy diet. It was usually the people who developed diabetes in their 60s and 70s who found it hardest to give up their taste for sweet things.'

The British Diabetic Association produces several recipe books ranging from everyday meals to delicious ideas for special occasions (see p 40). They show you how to make traditional favourites healthier, and also introduce some new recipes for you to try.

Different types of food

The food we eat falls into a number of different types, which do different jobs in the body. This section explains how to get the right balance between the different types of food.

Filling carbohydrates (starchy foods)

These are the foods that make us feel full and give us energy — foods such as potatoes, bread, pasta and rice. These foods are very important for people with diabetes because they are converted into glucose that enters the bloodstream. They are the starting point of the blood glucose level/insulin cycle (see p 5).

Some people with diabetes think that they should avoid starchy foods, because this idea was common in the past. In fact, completely the opposite is true. People with diabetes need regular amounts of carbohydrates (sometimes called CHOs) to help keep their blood glucose level steady.

High fibre carbohydrates

It is important to include some starchy foods that have not been refined, such as wholemeal bread and pasta, brown rice, jacket potatoes and wholemeal chapattis, as they contain much more fibre. They are good for people with diabetes, in fact they are good for everybody, because:

- they are more filling. This means they can help us lose weight;
- they help to prevent gut problems like constipation.

Not everyone likes these unrefined or 'whole' foods, so don't try to switch someone's diet dramatically overnight. It is best to introduce them gradually. For example you could try mixing wholemeal flour with white flour in baking or cooking. Or you could mix some wholemeal pasta in with plain pasta. Or you could leave the skins on potatoes when you cook them. But remember, you don't have to have 'brown' everything!

Carbohydrates as part of a diet for diabetes

Carbohydrates are so important for people with diabetes that every meal should contain some. The best way is to plan regular meals around starchy foods. For example cereals and/or toasted wholemeal bread are ideal for breakfast. For lunch and dinner you are spoiled for choice. You can choose between meals based on potatoes, rice, pasta, wholemeal bread, couscous or chappattis. You should be able to have your normal amount of starchy foods – but the dietitian can give you advice on spreading starchy foods over the day.

Sugars

Very sugary foods such as sweets and sugary soft drinks cause the blood glucose level to rise very quickly. These are the foods that, generally, people with diabetes should try to avoid – especially if they are overweight.

Mary

'I try to keep him away from the biscuit tin, but sometimes I notice it's gone down rather a lot. I try to keep a range of different biscuits in. And if I notice he's been at the biscuits, I try and get him to do some little jobs, like getting the vacuum out.'

If the person you care for has a very sweet tooth it's better not to try to cut these foods out altogether – it will only make them unhappy or tempt them to 'cheat'. It's better to encourage them to see sweet things as an occasional treat that they can enjoy without feeling guilty.

Here are some tips that may help the person you care for cut down on sugar:

- Always have plenty of fruit available, and encourage them to have a piece of fruit when they fancy something sweet.
- Choose the 'diet' or 'light' or 'slimline' versions of soft drinks and cordials – they contain artificial sweeteners which are both sugar and calorie free.
- Use artificial sweeteners such as Canderel, Hermesetas or Sweetex to sweeten tea or coffee. These are sometimes called 'intense' sweeteners. The BDA's *Sweetener Guide* explains the different kinds of sweeteners on the market.

■ Choose *unsweetened* tinned fruit and fruit juices.

■ Some puddings and desserts have low-sugar versions, eg sugar-free jelly (look out for 'diet' or 'light' or 'slimline' on the label).

■ Choose scones, tea cakes, currant loaf or malt loaf instead of rich cakes and pastries – these are lower in fat.

Having a sugary 'treat' as part of a meal will have less of an effect on blood glucose than having a sugary snack on an empty stomach. This is because the other foods will help to slow down the absorption of the sugar into the blood.

The recipe books produced by the British Diabetic Association (see p 40) are full of suggestions for cutting down on sugar and healthier eating for people with diabetes.

Eleanor

'As a young girl I did have quite a liking for sweet things, and I ate a lot of things that weren't good for me. But over the years I've cut down, and I've lost the desire now. It's taken me a long time to get to this point.'

What about special 'diabetic' foods?

Special 'diabetic' foods are confectionery foods with bulk sweeteners such as sorbitol or isomalt instead of sugar. They don't actually offer any special benefits for people with diabetes, they can be very expensive, and they sometimes cause diarrhoea and other digestive problems.

Annie

'One day Ernest had a bit of diarrhoea after breakfast. I gave him kaolin and morphine, but next day it happened again. I mentioned it to the nurse at the clinic, and she asked me what he was having for breakfast, then she told me to check my marmalade. It was special diabetic marmalade. When I read the label I saw it had sorbitol instead of sugar. "That'll be what's causing the diarrhoea," said the nurse, "It doesn't agree with everybody." She told me to use ordinary marmalade.'

Vegetables and fruit

Vegetables and fruit contain vitamins, minerals and fibre – all essential for a healthy diet. Eating more fruit and vegetables is associated with a reduced risk of a number of serious health problems, including cancer and heart disease. They help keep our skin, hair, teeth and bones healthy. And they help to shift the balance in what we eat to reduce calorie intake.

The good news is that someone with diabetes can eat as many vegetables and salads as they like. And there are countless new and interesting ways of preparing them. Even if you are not a vegetarian, vegetarian cookery books often have many unusual and appetising ideas for preparing vegetables.

If you are used to boiling vegetables, try saving the water for soups and stews so you get all the goodness from the vegetables. Or try cooking vegetables in the microwave with just a little water. Some vegetables are very tasty when baked or grilled.

The latest Government food guidelines suggest that everyone should try to eat at least five servings of fresh fruit or vegetables a day.

Fibre

Fibre is the part of plant foods that isn't broken down and digested in our stomach when we eat. People used to think that because fibre was not digested, it was no use to the human body. Now we know that fibre plays a very important part in helping our digestive system and our bowels to work properly. Fibre is important for people with diabetes because it helps slow down the rate at which glucose is absorbed by the body.

All plant foods contain fibre. Oats and pulse foods such as peas, beans and lentils, as well as some dried fruits and green vegetables, contain fibre which helps to control blood glucose level and also helps keep blood cholesterol down.

Foods with husks or bran, such as wholemeal flour and bread, brown pasta and brown rice, contain fibre which is good for preventing constipation.

However, some starchy foods which are not high fibre, like white pasta and basmati rice, are just as slowly absorbed and sustaining as high fibre versions. So you can enjoy a variety of starchy foods.

Proteins

Proteins are the foods that build the body up. Foods such as meat, fish, eggs and dairy products have a lot of protein. Some vegetables, especially nuts, beans and grains, contain protein too. Everybody needs a certain amount of protein, to help build and repair the cells of the body and to provide vital vitamins and minerals, but we all tend to eat too much protein these days.

Unfortunately meat and dairy foods also tend to contain a lot of fat. The healthy way to eat protein foods is to eat just a small portion, to trim off any visible fat from the meat, and to cook it without adding fat. Here are some suggestions for enjoying protein foods without too much fat:

- Trim visible fat off meat, and take the skin off chicken.
- Cut down on the size of the meat or fish portion. Fill up on extra starchy foods or vegetables instead.

- Try substituting vegetable proteins for meat proteins in some of your meals. For example soya products such as textured vegetable protein (TVP) are widely available, and you can use them instead of meat in many recipes. Or you could add extra tinned beans or lentils to casseroles and stews instead of meat.
- Try not to fry food — why not grill, roast, poach, steam, bake, braise, microwave, boil or stew it instead?
- While fish contains less fat than meat, oily fish contains fat but the fat it contains is better for you (but try to avoid frying it).
- Ready-made foods like sausages and burgers often contain a lot of fat. Look out for low-fat versions, and grill them instead of frying them.
- Use skimmed or semi-skimmed milk and choose low fat yoghurts.
- Go easy on cheese, or choose low-fat cheese, especially cottage cheese.

A closer look at fats and oils

Fats and oils give us energy, but they can also help to make us put on weight. We all tend to eat far more fat and oil than we need. For someone with diabetes (or for anyone) who needs to lose weight, the surest way is to cut down on the amount of fat and oil in the diet.

There are three kinds of fat. **Polyunsaturated fats** come mainly from vegetable oils such as sunflower and soya oil and are also found in fish. **Monounsaturated fats** are found mainly in olive oil and rapeseed oil. **Saturated fats** tend to come from meat or dairy products such as lard, butter, fatty meat, cheese and full fat milk.

All three types of fat contain a lot of calories, and make us put on weight. But in addition, **saturated fats** are linked with having high levels of cholesterol in the blood, which may contribute to heart disease. People with diabetes are at greater risk, so it makes sense to cut down on all fats, but particularly on saturated fats.

Many protein foods are high in fat, so follow the hints in the section above on proteins. In addition, you can cut down on fat by using low-fat spreads instead of butter or margarine – and spreading them very thinly.

If you do use fat for cooking, try to use monounsaturated oil, such as olive oil, or polyunsaturated oil, such as sunflower oil, instead of butter, margarine or lard. And try cutting down the amount you use.

Samina

'When my Dad found he had diabetes, we had to change the things we ate. We used to do all our cooking in ghee (a type of clarified butter). In our culture, using plenty of ghee is a sign of prosperity and status. But now we use olive or sunflower oil instead, and we limit the amount we use. Actually, I think the whole family is healthier as a result, and I prefer it. I use olive oil or sunflower oil for all my cooking now.'

Salt

High salt intake has been linked to high blood pressure. People with diabetes are more at risk if they have high blood pressure (see Chapter 6) so it makes sense to reduce the amount of salt in the diet.

There are four main ways to cut down on salt:

- Add less salt when you are cooking – use other flavourings like herbs and spices.
- Cut down on salted foods like crisps and nuts.
- Eat fewer tinned, processed, ready-prepared or smoked foods.
- Don't add salt to your plate.

If you cut down the amount of salt gradually, it will be much less noticeable than if you try to stop using salt suddenly. Try experimenting with more herbs, spices and lemon juice in cooking instead of salt. Everyday herbs such as parsley, and everyday spices such as black pepper can be just as tasty as the more exotic varieties.

Alcohol

Having an occasional alcoholic drink does no harm so long as it's taken sensibly. Too much alcohol, or drinking alcohol on an empty stomach, isn't good for any of us, and can cause a 'hypo' in someone with diabetes who is on tablets or insulin, because alcohol lowers the blood glucose level -- and the effects of the alcohol may make them unaware that a 'hypo' is coming on. (See Chapter 8 for more about 'hypos'.)

Sensible drinking means:

- never drinking on an empty stomach, or skipping a meal to have a drink instead;
- having a good snack before going to bed if you have had a drink in the evening;
- limiting alcohol to three units a day for men, and two units a day for women, or 28 units a week for men, and 21 units a week for women (a unit is roughly equal to half a pint of beer or a glass of wine or a single measure of spirit);
- trying to have some days when you have no alcohol at all.

Note If you are taking any medication, check with your doctor, nurse or pharmacist whether the alcohol limits are the same.

Alcoholic drinks also tend to be high in calories -- a problem if someone is trying to lose weight. Low sugar 'diet' beers and lagers tend to be high in alcohol, while low-alcohol drinks and soft drinks are often high in sugar. Look out for low alcohol beers and lagers that are also low in sugar. If the person you care for has a favourite drink, ask the doctor or the nurse at the clinic how much it is safe for them to have. You may need to take an empty bottle or can along so that they can read the label.

Marie

'My husband used to be a big drinker – a nine-pints-a-night man. In the day he worked on the kilns, so he got very thirsty, and he would always have four spoonfuls of sugar in his tea. Now he's dropped all his bad habits, drinking, sugar, even smoking – he gave up just like that.'

For more *i*nformation

ℹ *Alcohol and diabetes* published by the British Diabetic Association.

Planning healthy meals

The dietitian will help you to plan a healthy diet for the person you care for. A quick guide is the diagram below. The plate of food should look like this:

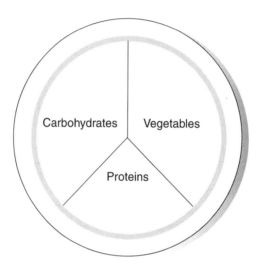

Keith

'Val used to do the cooking, but now she's had her legs amputated I've taken over. I did cook at home when I was a boy, so I'm used to it, but now I'm getting a bit more adventurous. I like to try out the new recipes in *Balance* (the BDA magazine) – and I know what we can and can't have. We always have two or three vegetables as well as potatoes and meat, and if possible a Yorkshire pudding. We never bother with the special diabetic foods or jams at all.'

Fasting at Ramadan

During the month of Ramadan, most Muslims fast between sunrise and sunset. People who are unwell or have certain conditions, including diabetes, do not have to fast, but many still choose to fast if they can.

If someone is taking insulin, it is best not to fast, as going for a long time without food can cause the blood glucose level to fall too low and bring on a 'hypo'. If someone is trying to control his or her diabetes with diet, it may be possible to observe the fast, but it is best to get specific advice from your doctor, nurse or dietitian. If someone is taking tablets then they should discuss with their doctor whether they can go without taking their tablets or any food at all during the daylight hours.

Much depends on when Ramadan falls in any particular year. If Ramadan falls in the winter, the fast may only be for eight hours or so. People can change their medication and eating times so they are still getting as much food in the non-fasting period. But if Ramadan falls in the summer, it may mean going for eighteen hours without anything to eat or drink. This makes it much harder to control blood glucose level.

People with diabetes can be exempted from fasting without breaking with their religion. It is up to the individual to discuss with their doctor how fasting might affect their diabetes and weigh up the reasons for fasting against the possible risks.

Samina

'My Dad has been controlling his diabetes just through watching his diet, and in the past he has always managed to observe the Ramadan fast. But this year he decided not to fast. For one thing he's started taking tablets to control his diabetes. Also, he has been quite unwell, and hasn't got over an infection he picked up. So although this year it is a winter Ramadan, which is much easier, he decided not to observe the fast. He's a very religious man, but I'm glad he's been sensible and I'm sure it was the right decision.'

For more *i*nformation

i If you need help or advice about choosing the right diet for the person you care for, ask your doctor or the nurse at the clinic, or ask to see the dietitian.

i The British Diabetic Association have a Diet Information Service. See 'Useful Addresses' or ring their *Careline* on 0171-636 6112.

i The British Diabetic Association also have a large selection of information leaflets and recipe books, including:

Food Choices and Diabetes;

Everyday cookery – healthy recipes for the older person;

Eating well with diabetes;

Healthy Asian cookery.

There is a charge for most of these. To find out the current cost and how to order, contact the British Diabetic Association Distribution Department (address on p 124).

Healthy living

Making sure that the person you care for is eating a healthy diet is important, but it's not the only thing that matters. A healthy lifestyle also means being the right weight for your height, getting enough exercise, and above all it means cutting out cigarettes.

Losing weight

More than three out of four people with type 2 diabetes are overweight. Your dietitian will advise you, but even losing a small amount of weight can help you to manage your diabetes more easily.

Being overweight makes blood glucose control more difficult, and it's also bad for the heart. So if the person you care for has been told to lose some weight, here's how you can help:

- Don't encourage any 'crash' diets. They are hard to keep to, and so they don't work in the long term. Remember, the diet that really works is the one that can be kept up for months – and years. Encourage the person you care for to lose weight gradually. That way the weight will come off slowly and will stay off.
- Make sure the person eats regularly, and help them plan what they will eat at each meal – that way they will have something to look forward to, and will feel less tempted to 'snack'.
- Have plenty of fruit in the house, so that if they do fancy a snack they can have something that is good for them. Buy wholemeal bread or crackers, or oatcakes, instead of sweets and biscuits. If the person you care for likes to 'raid the fridge' from time to time, make sure they will find tempting healthy salads with low-fat dressing, low-fat yoghurts and cottage cheese. Keeping a 'store' of sugary treats and sweets is a sure way to encourage temptation.
- Follow the healthy eating guidelines on pages 27–40. Remember: DO avoid fatty foods and trim the fat off meat.

  DO choose 'low fat', 'diet', 'light' or 'lite' options when they are available as they can help you cut down on calories.

  DO choose skimmed or semi-skimmed milk, yoghurt and low-fat cheese.

  DO go easy on alcoholic drinks – alcohol is high in calories and therefore very fattening. It also stimulates appetite.

  DON'T fry food – grill, bake, microwave or boil instead.

  DON'T buy crisps, sweets, cakes, nuts or biscuits regularly – save them for an occasional treat.

  DON'T waste your money on special 'diabetic' foods – they have the same calories as standard foods.

  DON'T be tempted by special 'meal replacement' foods for slimmers – they only work in the short term.
- If someone is trying to lose weight, they should weigh themselves regularly at the same time each week and make a note of the reading. That will help build up a long-term picture of which way their weight is going. Reading weight more often can be misleading, as our weight fluctuates daily and throughout the day.
- Make sure the person you care for is getting enough exercise (there is more about this in the next section).

- If the person you care for is still finding it difficult to lose weight, book them in to see the dietitian, and go along with them. The dietitian will take a closer look at what they are eating every day, and suggest changes to help reduce their calorie intake.
- Losing weight is never easy, so make sure the person has plenty of ongoing support to help them keep to their new healthy eating habits.
- Remember that small, maintainable changes are all that is generally needed.

Getting enough exercise

Getting enough exercise is important for many reasons:

- Exercise tones up all the muscles – it helps an older person stay active and independent.
- It strengthens the heart muscle, giving protection against heart disease.
- It burns up calories, so it can help someone to lose weight.
- It is a very effective way of warding off depression.
- Some forms of exercise, such as dancing, aquarobics or classes at the local leisure centre are a good way of getting out and about and meeting new friends.
- Exercise burns up blood glucose, so exercising regularly helps keep the blood glucose levels stable. This is especially important if someone is trying to control their diabetes with diet.
- Exercise can make the body use insulin or tablets more efficiently.
- It improves circulation and helps prevent nerve damage.
- Regular exercise can lower blood pressure.
- It can protect against osteoporosis (thinning of the bones, leading to fractures, which is common especially among older women).

With ten good reasons like these, you should be able to persuade the person you care for to take more exercise – but perhaps the main reason is just that it will make them feel better – both physically and mentally.

Exercise for older people

Older people are often reluctant to take exercise because they think it has to be something strenuous like running the marathon or jumping up and down to loud music. In fact the aim should be just to get slightly out of breath, and have a pleasant warm 'glow'. If they are feeling pain or panting for breath then they are overdoing it!

Or maybe they don't want to be bothered with special clothing or equipment or having to go somewhere at a regular time. Some people like to join a club or a class, but exercise needn't mean special 'gear' or even leaving the home. It is just as easy to build regular exercise into the daily routine.

The important thing is to build up slowly. Even gentle exercise, such as hoovering or polishing or walking up the stairs, can get the heart beating a little faster. Then they should build up step by step, until they are walking briskly, gardening, dancing, cycling or swimming for at least 20 minutes a day, five days a week.

Exercise for people with diabetes

Exercise helps lower the blood glucose level. If someone is already taking tablets or insulin to reduce their blood glucose level, they may need less when they start taking exercise. It is important if someone is on insulin or tablets to test the blood glucose level more regularly when they first start exercising, because if it falls too low the result could be a 'hypo' (see Chapter 8).

Exercise for people with a disability

Even people who have disabilities or arthritis or who are in a wheelchair can benefit from 'armchair' exercises. Moving and stretching arms, legs and neck can help keep joints supple and gently exercise the heart. Some local authorities and health authorities put on special exercise classes for people with disabilities.

Swimming is another form of exercise which is excellent for many people with disabilities. Many leisure centres run special groups for older or disabled swimmers, and some may even warm the water up specially – very relaxing!

> ### Val
>
> 'Some people think just because you've got diabetes you're an invalid, but you don't have to be. Since I lost my legs two years ago, I can't do as much, but I still try to keep active. I can't do the garden anymore, Keith does that, but I can still do the window boxes.'

For more *i*nformation

i You can find out about exercise videos or exercise classes aimed at older people from Age Concern England (address on page 132) or from your local clinic.

i Age Concern Factsheet 45 *Fitness for Later Life* which is full of ideas and information about fitness and exercise for older people.

Time to stop smoking

It is never easy to persuade someone to stop smoking. It's something each person has to decide for themselves. But if the person you care for is a smoker, then being diagnosed with diabetes gives them the best reason in the world to stop. Smoking narrows the blood vessels, so it makes complications such as heart disease, nerve damage leading to amputation, eye problems and kidney disease all much more likely.

If you are a smoker yourself, you can help the person you care for to stop smoking by not offering them cigarettes and not smoking in front of them. (You could use this opportunity to give up smoking yourself!)

If you are a non-smoker yourself, it may be better to get professional help. You may find it difficult to understand the person's craving for cigarettes. And they may resent being told what to do by you.

The doctor or the nurse at the clinic will have already suggested giving up smoking. Ask them for their advice, and find out about aids such as nicotine patches or nicotine chewing gum, which can help ease the craving for a cigarette.

For more *i*nformation

i **Quitline** is a national helpline for people who want to stop smoking. They can tell you about stop-smoking groups in your area and give you advice and encouragement. You will get through to a trained volunteer during office hours, or a recorded message outside these times. Phone them on Quitline: 0800 00 22 00.

4 Taking tablets to control diabetes

About half of all people with type 2 diabetes can control their diabetes with tablets, backed up by a healthy diet. The tablets are called oral antidiabetics, because they are taken by mouth (oral) and control the amount of glucose in the blood. Some tablets work by stimulating the pancreas to produce more insulin, so they are only suitable for people who are still able to produce some insulin (this includes most people who develop diabetes in later life). Other drugs enable the insulin produced to work more effectively, and some slow down the speed at which glucose is absorbed by the body.

Joe

'I used to just take two tablets a day, but when they put it up to five, I found it hard to remember which tablets I'd taken, so I worked out a system that helps me remember. I have to take Glipizide with breakfast and at teatime. They come in strips of two, so that's easy – if there's one left, it means I haven't taken one. I have to take Metformin three times a day, with breakfast, dinner and at teatime. I saved an old Metformin bottle, and I put three tablets in it each morning. Then I can see how many I've taken and how many I still have to take. I watched the nurses when I was in hospital, and that's how they did it.'

Different types of tablets

Every person with diabetes is different, with a different medical history and different lifestyle, so the doctor will try to work out an individual programme for each person. Many people with diabetes take a combination of tablets to help them maintain a healthy blood glucose level throughout the day. The dose and timing of tablets can therefore be quite complicated.

If you are caring for someone with diabetes, you will probably find it useful to know both the generic name (that is, the *type* of tablets) and the brand name of the tablets that have been prescribed for them.

Sulphonylureas

Sulphonylureas were first discovered in the 1950s and since then have been taken successfully by many thousands of people. They work mainly by stimulating the cells in the pancreas to make more insulin, and also by helping the insulin to work more effectively. The table on the next page shows the most common sulphonylureas.

Many doctors like to prescribe tablets they are familiar with, often ones which have been in use for a long time such as Glibenclamide. But there are other factors the doctor will take into account.

Sulphonylurea tablets are usually given to people who are not very overweight, as they have a tendency to cause weight increase. Tablets such as Glibenclamide which are long-acting only need to be taken once a day and the effect lasts up to 18 hours. This can be an advantage for someone who is forgetful about taking tablets, but it can also cause problems. It is important for anyone taking these long-acting tablets to eat meals with carbohydrate regularly, otherwise their blood glucose level can become dangerously low. (This is called having a 'hypo' and it is described more fully in Chapter 8). Other sulphonylurea tablets, such as Tolbutamide,

47

The most common sulphonylureas

Generic name	Brand name	When taken	Action
Glibenclamide	Daonil, Euglucon, Semi Daonil	Divided dose before meals, or daily with breakfast	Long-acting
Gliclazide	Diamicron	Divided dose with main meals or daily with breakfast	Medium-acting
Glipizide	Minodiab, Glibenese	Before meals	Medium-acting
Gliquidone	Glurenorm	Before meals	Short-acting
Tolbutamide	Rastinon	With or before meals	Short-acting
Tolazamide	Tolanase	With breakfast	Medium-acting

Gliquidone or Glicazide, act more quickly and need to be taken with or before meals to be effective.

Whatever tablets are prescribed, it's very important for someone with diabetes to keep to instructions about meal times to avoid the risk of a 'hypo'. If the person you are caring for doesn't eat regularly or sometimes gets confused about mealtimes, you should discuss this with their doctor.

Possible side effects

The most serious side effect of these tablets can be having a 'hypo', when the blood glucose drops dangerously low. 'Hypo', short for hypoglycaemia, is discussed more fully in Chapter 8. Other side effects can include an upset stomach, nausea and headache.

Extra care is needed when older people or people with liver and kidney problems take sulphonylureas, because of the risk of hypoglycaemia. People who have other conditions as well as diabetes, or who are taking other medicines, may also experience side effects.

Other drugs, including sulphonamide antibiotics, probenecid, anti-coagulants including warfarin, beta-blockers, chloramphenicol, monamine oxidase inhibitors, sulphinpyrazone, phenylbutazone and even aspirin can interact with sulphonylureas, lowering blood glucose levels and causing a 'hypo'. As many of these are quite common drugs, taken by thousands of older people, it is important to be on the lookout for the possible side effects. Some older people are prescribed a small daily dose of aspirin after they have had a stroke. This dose is too low to affect their blood glucose level.

If you buy any medicines over the counter, always tell the pharmacist if they are for someone with diabetes, or check with your doctor first. The doctor should always be informed about other medicines someone is taking.

Biguanides

The only biguanide used in this country is Metformin. Metformin works by stopping the liver from producing new glucose, and by making insulin carrying glucose into muscle and cells work more effectively. Like sulphonylureas, they only work for people who are still producing some insulin of their own. Metformin is often prescribed for people who are overweight as it is not associated with weight gain. It will also not normally cause a 'hypo', unless it is taken with sulphonylureas. However, it can have some unpleasant side effects, so it is not suitable for everyone. It is very important that the doctor is aware if the person you care for has had any kidney or liver problems, or has a condition affecting their heart or their circulation.

There is only one biguanide prescribed in this country, but it comes under a number of different brand names:

Generic name	Brand name	When taken	Action
Metformin	Glucophage Metformin	With or after meals	Short-acting

Possible side effects

Many people get an upset stomach when they first start taking Metformin. They may feel queasy and lose their appetite, or they may even get diarrhoea. This is not serious and usually settles down after a few weeks. Sometimes the doctor will reduce the dose of the drug until the problem settles down.

Some people who take Metformin may also, very rarely, get lactic acidosis. This is when waste acids build up in the blood causing severe cramps. It is more likely to happen in people over 65, people who have kidney or liver damage, or who drink a lot of alcohol. Lactic acidosis can be serious, especially in people with chest or heart problems. If the person you are caring for has been prescribed Metformin tablets (Glucophage or Metformin) do keep the doctor informed about any side effects.

Alpha-glucosidase inhibitors

These tablets help to keep blood glucose levels down by blocking the absorption of carbohydrates in the intestine. They must be taken with food – either swallowed whole with some liquid just before a meal, or chewed with the first mouthful. These tablets work on the digestive system rather than on the insulin cycle, and they are sometimes given to people who are overweight and who have tried without success to control their diabetes just with diet.

Generic name	Brand name	When Taken	Action
Acarbose	Glucobay	With a meal	Short-acting

Possible side effects

They do not lead to 'hypos', but they can cause wind, stomach rumbling and diarrhoea at first. Let the doctor know if these symptoms have not settled down in two to three weeks. As with Metformin, 'hypos' can occur if Acarbose is taken with a sulphonylurea.

Why it is important to take tablets regularly

Tablets can be very effective at controlling blood glucose level but only if they are taken regularly. Sometimes an older person with diabetes may be confused or forgetful about meals and medication. If you are caring for someone like this, try to establish a simple routine of eating meals and taking tablets that is easy to remember and stick to.

- If you live with the person you care for and are at home with them most of the day, you can plan regular meals and between-meals snacks, and make sure tablets are taken at the right time.

- If you see the person every day, you could prepare or buy meals that only need heating up, and you could use an alarm clock or a timer to remind them of meal times and times for taking tablets. You can buy special tablet dispensing boxes with labelled compartments for all the tablets to be taken (ask the chemist).

- If you are caring for someone at a distance you may be able to plan meals weekly in advance, and set up a system of alarm reminders. You (or someone reliable) can set out the tablets once a week using a tablet-dispensing box which you can get from the chemist. Some boxes have a separate section for each day of the week as well as compartments for morning, afternoon and evening. You may be able to stock up the freezer with pre-prepared meals or use a delivery service such as meals on wheels.

- However, if this doesn't work, you may need to arrange for someone to call round at regular times. A neighbour, friend or relative might be willing to do this, but if not, ask social services for help. They can arrange for someone to call round in the morning to set out the tablets in the box, and perhaps call later in the day as well. Sometimes an arrangement like this may be all that is needed to keep someone living at home rather than needing to go into residential care. (There is more about help from social services in Chapter 9).

What to do if you forget a tablet

Everyone forgets to take their medication from time to time. If this happens and its only an hour or two since the normal time for taking the tablet, then it should be taken as soon as it is remembered. If it is longer than a couple of hours, the best thing is to miss the dose altogether and take the next tablet at the normal time. It can be dangerous to take two tablets instead of one, as it can lower the blood glucose level too much.

If you find that the person you care for is forgetting meals or tablets quite often, it is important to talk to their doctor. It may be possible to simplify the number of tablets they are taking or to find other ways to make sure they take their tablets regularly.

Taking tablets during illness

Someone who is ill still needs to take their tablets regularly to keep their blood glucose level stable. Some tablets need to be taken with food, and if the person you care for is feeling off their food or cannot eat a meal you should encourage them to have some soup or milk or fruit juice with their tablets instead.

If the person is vomiting or has diarrhoea, they may not be absorbing the tablets and their blood glucose level may start to go up. If this happens, contact the GP or diabetes clinic immediately. Some infections can also cause the blood glucose level to rise. If someone is ill, they should check their blood glucose levels at least four times a day. If the levels start to rise, contact the GP or the diabetic clinic at once. The doctor may advise having insulin injections temporarily until the illness settles down.

Moving from tablets to insulin

Some people can control their diabetes for a while by taking tablets and eating a healthy diet, but as time goes by their blood glucose level starts to rise again. This may show up in their regular blood or urine tests, or the first signs may be that they start to feel tired and unwell. If this happens, let the doctor know. Sometimes changing the amount or type of tablets can be enough to stabilise the blood glucose level, but sometimes the doctor will recommend insulin injections.

Not everyone who has insulin injections has to have them for the rest of their life. If the rise in blood glucose level is due to illness (see above) then it may be possible to go back to tablets once the illness is over. But about 25 to 30 per cent of people with type 2 diabetes do control their diabetes with insulin injections.

The thought of having to give themselves regular injections can be frightening or distasteful to some people. No one can pretend that it is an easy or pleasant thing to do. But in fact people often say that thinking about it is much worse than doing it. Usually, the person starts to feel so much better that they realise it is worth it.

There is more about controlling diabetes with insulin in the next chapter.

Carolyn

Carolyn is a diabetes specialist nurse in Sheffield.

'We've been carrying out some trials, offering suitable people with type 2 diabetes insulin for six months and then, where appropriate, giving them the option of going back onto tablets. But in our pilot study, not one person chose to go back onto tablets.'

Audrey

'At first, when they told me I had to have injections, I said no way can I shove a needle into my stomach or into my arm. They gave me some new innovation – a gun thing – but I couldn't work it. The district nurse came and did it for me. Even when I went away on holiday I had to arrange for the district nurse to come out and give me my injections. Then I said to myself, this is a fool's game. Other people do it, why can't I do it? Now I don't even think about it. It's just part of my daily routine.'

For more *i*nformation

ℹ Ask your pharmacist, your GP or your specialist diabetes nurse if you are unsure about anything to do with taking tablets.

ℹ *Treating diabetes with tablets* and *Living with diabetes for those treated with diet and tablets* published by the British Diabetic Association.

5 Treating diabetes with insulin

Since insulin was discovered in 1921, it has saved the lives of thousands of people with diabetes. Both people with type 1 diabetes (Insulin Dependent Diabetes Mellitus) and people with type 2 diabetes (Non-Insulin Dependent Diabetes Mellitus) can use insulin as part of their treatment. This chapter looks at the different kinds of insulin and at how they are used.

Eleanor

'I'm a great believer in natural remedies, so I tried for a long time to control my diabetes with diet. I hated the thought of injections. I tried herbal treatments, and I tried acupuncture. But I just got worse and worse. I felt tired all the time, and I was losing weight. After they put me on tablets I still carried on losing weight. In two years I went down from 11 stone to 7½ stone. In the end they took me into hospital and put me on insulin. I felt better instantly.

'Now I wish I'd started on the insulin earlier. I don't think I'd have had all the trouble with my eyes.'

Insulin injections for people with diabetes

Insulin is a protein that is digested and broken down in the stomach. At present it is not possible to take insulin orally – it has to be injected. Scientists have found ways of coating insulin or treating it so that it can be taken in orally, but they are now working to discover an accurate way of assessing dosage, as insulin is absorbed differently through the stomach.

The thought of having lots of injections is so worrying to some people that they try to avoid taking insulin for as long as possible. In the past, insulin injections were quite painful, as the needles were larger and had to be slid in under the skin. Older people may have known friends or relatives who had to inject insulin using the older type of needles, and may have unpleasant memories.

Nowadays the needles are very fine and short, or people can use a special injecting 'pen' with a ready-filled cartridge. People who do start to take insulin often wish they had started much sooner.

Different types of insulin

In the past, all insulin given to people with diabetes used to come from pork or beef. The pancreas was taken from the animals when they were slaughtered for other purposes. Many people have used porcine or bovine insulin successfully for years. However, the body recognises that animal insulin is slightly different to human insulin produced naturally. It sometimes causes reactions in people such as itching, bumps or redness around the injection site, but this is quite rare.

Nowadays most people take 'human' insulin. Human insulin does not come from human pancreases. Scientists have discovered a way in which to engineer certain types of bacteria to produce insulin that is identical to human insulin. This allows for large amounts of purified 'human' insulin to be produced. However, animal insulin is still available for people who prefer it.

Some people who switched from animal insulin to human insulin found they were having 'hypos' more often and more severely. The warning signs they had learnt to recognise, to tell them that a hypo was coming on, didn't seem to be working. No one is sure why this happens. However, most people who switch from animal to human insulin notice no difference at all.

Val

Val was one of the first people to use the new human insulin. 'It's quite a bit keener than the beef insulin I'd been using before. I had two "hypos" without any warning. Once I passed out in the street. They took me off it and put me back on beef insulin. But then I thought that maybe it was other things, such as the change of life that I was going through, that had made me lose some of my warning signs. They put me back on human insulin for a second time, and I had no problems. They gradually reduced my dose. Now I'm on less insulin than when I was first diagnosed, and I've got my warning signs back.'

Doctors now think that most people with diabetes do better on human insulin. If someone is starting to take insulin for the first time the doctor will generally prescribe them human insulin.

Short-, medium- and long-acting insulins

Some insulins act very rapidly to remove glucose from the blood, while others are more long-acting, and give background protection all day. Many people use both types at different times or in combination.

If the person you care for is using insulin, their doctor or specialist nurse will work out a combination of types of insulin to suit both their lifestyle and their medical needs. You may have to mix the insulin yourself, or you may be able to buy it ready-mixed.

Short-acting insulin

Short-acting insulin is also known as soluble insulin. It is a clear, colourless liquid. It works quickly to lower the blood glucose. It is normally taken 15-30 minutes before a meal to cover the rise in blood glucose that occurs after eating. It has a peak action within two to six hours after injecting and it can last up to eight hours.

If it appears cloudy, discoloured or lumpy, it should not be used.

Medium- and long-acting insulins

These insulins act over a period of up to 30 hours, and help to control blood glucose level between meals. Their peak activity is usually four to twelve hours after injection. They are usually taken once or twice a day to provide an even background level of insulin. Sometimes short-acting insulin is also taken to cope with the extra glucose absorbed during meals.

These insulins have chemicals added to slow down their action, so they look white and cloudy. When the bottle has been standing for a while the cloudiness may settle into a layer at the bottom – this is normal. However, the cloudiness should be even. If there are lumps or clumps floating in the bottle, do not use it.

Analogue insulin

This is a new type of insulin made by altering the insulin molecule to make it even faster-acting. It can be injected with or just after a meal and lasts between two and five hours. Often people take it with another longer-acting type of insulin that controls blood glucose level between meals.

This insulin is clear, and unlike other short-acting insulins, it does not go cloudy when it is 'off'. Instead you may see 'frosting' round the bottle or particles in the insulin. If this happens, don't use it.

Scientists are trying to create other types of analogue insulin that work at different speeds.

Getting the right combination of insulins

With so many different types of insulin available, the doctor or specialist nurse can choose a treatment to take into account both someone's medical needs and their preferences and life-style. People respond differently to the different types of insulin available. They may act more quickly, or more slowly, in some people than others. For some people, one injection of a medium- or long-acting insulin may be enough, while others will take a combination of short- and long-acting insulins. Some people choose to mix their own insulins, or the carer may mix the insulins for them. Others buy their insulins already mixed. If the person you care for has any problems with the insulin they are taking, a different type or combination may suit them better, so let the doctor or specialist nurse know.

Injecting insulin

Sometimes the carer may need to learn how to give insulin injections, but more often the person with diabetes learns how to inject the insulin.

Keith and Val

Keith does Val's injections for her when she is ill. 'Val prefers to do her own injections, but when she's not very well, I do it for her. It's much better with the new injection pens – I couldn't do it with the old needles they used to use.'

Injecting with a syringe

Some people use an ordinary syringe, and draw the insulin up from a glass bottle. If someone is taking a mixture of insulins which is not sold in cartridges, then they will need to mix the insulin in the syringe.

The doctor or diabetes specialist nurse will show you how to draw the insulin.

1   Long- and medium-acting insulins have a cloudy layer that settles on the bottom of the bottle. Before you inject, make sure the insulin is well-mixed by rotating it or turning it upside down several times (but do not shake it vigorously).

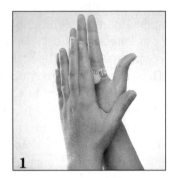

2   Draw air up into the syringe (the same amount as the number of units you want to inject).

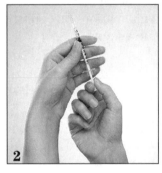

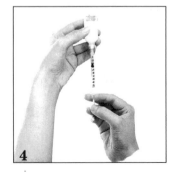

3   Inject the air through the rubber seal into the bottle of insulin. (Not all doctors and nurses think steps 2 and 3 are necessary.)

4   With the needle still in the bottle, turn the bottle upside down, so the syringe is at the bottom, and gently draw the insulin down into the syringe to the correct amount.

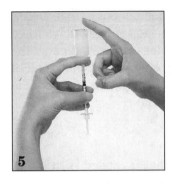

5 Remove any bubbles by holding the syringe needle-upwards and tapping gently till the bubble floats up to the needle. Then push the plunger in a little way to force the bubble out. The bubbles are not harmful, but they reduce the amount of insulin in the syringe.

6 Now gently remove the syringe from the bottle, and you are ready to inject.

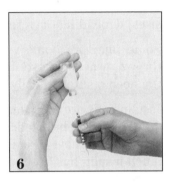

If you are mixing insulin in the syringe, you need to go through these steps with both insulins, drawing up the clear insulin before the cloudy.

The syringes come in three sizes, depending on the amount of insulin you are taking: 1 ml (100 units); 0.5 ml (50 units); 0.3 ml (30 units). The syringe needles are also available in varying lengths. The injection technique you use affects the length of needle you should choose – your diabetes care team will be able to help you. These are available on prescription. The needles used to inject insulin are very fine, so they don't hurt much, and they are

Source: Reproduced by kind permission of Becton Dickinson UK Limited, taken from their booklet 'Getting Started with Diabetes'.

very short because the injections are subcutaneous – that means they are given just below the skin, so the needle doesn't have to go in very deep. It is also possible to buy devices which will inject the needle automatically. The needle goes into the skin at the touch of a button. These are not available on prescription, but if you would like to try using one, ask at your diabetic clinic.

Using a pen injector

Many people use a special pen injector that is loaded with a cartridge of insulin. Pen injectors are supplied by the manufacturers of insulin cartridges and come free of charge from the diabetic clinic. The needles have to be bought separately and come in three sizes, depending on your body size.

Some injectors come ready-loaded with the cartridges and are thrown away after use. You can also buy pen injectors that release the needle automatically at the touch of a button.

Insulin pens are often much better for people with arthritis as they do not need to be filled. And they may help people with poor eyesight as they have a dial on the end which 'clicks' to indicate how much insulin has been taken and how much is left.

Eleanor

'I use a NovoPen. I find it very convenient, and I hardly think about it anymore. There's a little raised dial that clicks round at the end so I can count how much I've had, and how much I've still got to take. It's ideal for me because I've had a lot of trouble with my eyesight. I didn't think I'd ever get used to injecting myself, but now it's just part of my daily routine.'

Other injection systems

You may have heard of *jet injectors*, which deliver a stream of insulin under very high pressure straight through the skin. Some people prefer them because they don't use needles, but the high pressure can cause bruising on the skin if they are not used with great care. They are not available on the NHS and are not available or widely used in the UK, but if you would like to consider using one talk to your doctor or nurse at the diabetes clinic.

An *insulin pump* works by sending a continuous flow of insulin into your body through a fine needle. It is worn next to the body, and the needle has to be changed every day. Again, these are quite expensive and not available on the NHS but your doctor or the nurse at the clinic will be able to advise you.

How to inject insulin

Many people with diabetes prefer to inject themselves, but if you need to inject the person you care for, the way to do it is quickly and smoothly.

Choose a part of the body that has plenty of fat beneath the skin. The upper arms, thighs, buttocks and stomach are all good places to inject (the doctor or specialist nurse will show you where to inject). The needle should go in at a right angle (90°) into the fatty tissue beneath the skin. If the person has been advised to pinch up the skin, they should do so – but do not pinch the skin up too firmly as this will make the injection more painful.

Make sure the skin is clean before you inject, but there is no need to swab with alcohol. Sometimes you may notice a small spot of blood or insulin after taking out the needle. This is nothing to worry about. Just press lightly on the spot with a clean finger or with a clean piece of cotton wool for a few moments.

Sometimes you may notice that a small amount of insulin is leaking out from the skin after you have withdrawn the needle. If this happens, it is a good idea to give an extra blood test after the meal. But don't give a second injection to try to make up the amount of insulin that has been lost. If you find this leakage is happening regularly, ask your doctor or specialist nurse for advice about your injection technique.

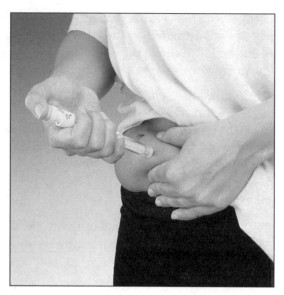

The first few times you inject someone it may hurt more, because both you and the person being injected are feeling nervous and tense. As you get more practice your technique will improve, and the person you are injecting will get more used to it, too.

Val

'When I first started injecting myself, they let me practice a few times on an orange. Then the day came and they said, "Right, you've got to do it yourself." I sat on the edge of my bed and cried. The needles were much thicker in those days, and you had to slide it in under the skin. Nowadays, you just stick it in. It's nothing, really, compared to how it was.'

Problems with injecting

Lumps and bumps

If you inject too often in the same place, lumps or bruising may appear under the skin. It is important to rotate the injection sites so that each area has time to recover. You can inject several times into each of the injection areas before moving on to another area (eg left arm, right arm, left leg, right leg, stomach, left buttock, right buttock) but don't put the needle in exactly the same place as this will affect the absorption. Keep a chart or reminder — don't just rely on memory.

Blunt needles

Many people use plastic disposable syringes or pens more than once, but if the needle is blunt or bent, throw it away. Using a blunt needle makes injections more painful.

Leakage

Sometimes the insulin doesn't all go where you want it to go — a little of it may leak out after the needle has been withdrawn. If this happens, monitor the blood glucose level carefully to make sure that the person has had sufficient insulin, but don't give an extra dose. If it happens regularly, mention it to the doctor or the diabetes specialist nurse. You may need some help with your injection technique.

Some possible effects of insulin

Speed of action

Sometimes the insulin acts more quickly than usual. This can happen if the skin is very warm (for instance if the person has a hot bath or sits in the sun). Physical exercise can also speed up the action of insulin – for example, if someone runs after injecting into the leg, or does housework after an injection into the upper arm, the insulin will work faster. Massaging the injection area can make insulin work faster too.

Blurred vision

Some people find their eyesight changes after they start taking insulin. This is because high glucose levels cause the lens in the eye to change shape slightly. As diabetes control improves it usually corrects itself. Put off getting new glasses until your diabetes control is stable. Ask the GP or diabetes care team for advice.

Weight gain

Some people may put weight on when they start to take insulin. This can be a positive sign, as weight loss is often a symptom of poor diabetes control. But putting on too much weight can be unhealthy, so try to cut down on high-fat foods on a regular basis such as fried foods and full-fat dairy products, and follow the guidelines on healthy eating in Chapter 3. If the person you are caring for is having a lot of snacks, because they are worried about going 'hypo', make sure that plenty of low-fat foods which contain carbohydrate are available, such as fruit or crispbread, and talk about the problem with your health care team.

Disposing of needles

Never throw used needles or syringes in the bin. It is very easy for someone to injure themselves. Ask at the clinic what is the best way of disposing of used needles.

Some hospitals and clinics have a collection point for used needles. It is often called a 'sharps box'.

If you have to dispose of the needles yourself, you can get a special needle clipper on prescription. This will snap the needles off your syringe or pen and keep them safely in an enclosed container. When it is full (it should hold about 200 needles) you can simply throw it away in the bin. Put used syringes and lancets in a hard plastic container such as a margarine tub or detergent bottle with a child-proof lid, and throw them in the bin (make sure the point of the lancet is pressed well into the cover). General guidelines should be followed with agreement from your local authority refuse department.

Looking after your insulin

The best place to keep insulin is in the fridge. But keep it well away from the freezer compartment. Insulin that has been frozen is not safe to use.

If you can't keep insulin in the fridge, the next best place is a cool dark spot such as a drawer.

It is safe to keep insulin at room temperature for up to one month, so long as it is not warmer than 25° centigrade or 70° Fahrenheit. But never leave it near a cooker, radiator or heater nor on top of electrical equipment such as a TV, computer or music centre. On warm days, make sure the insulin is not left in bright sunlight, and never leave it in the car, where it can get very hot.

If you are travelling, you can keep insulin cool in a cool-bag, or a wide-necked vacuum flask, or you can buy special insulated containers. When you travel by air, don't forget to keep the insulin with you in your hand baggage.

Always use the insulin before the expiry date. Once a vial has been opened, use it within the specified time, which is usually 28 days, or throw it away.

Hazel

'My Mum's 80 and she needs a lot of care. But she still gives herself injections every day. She's brilliant.'

For more *i*nformation

ⓘ Ask your pharmacist, your GP or your specialist diabetes nurse if you are unsure about anything to do with using insulin.

ⓘ Leaflets produced by the British Diabetic Association, including: *Insulin*; *Storing your own insulin*; *Changing from tablets to insulin* and *The Insulin Debate*.

6 Diabetes and other health problems

This chapter looks at some of the complications that can arise with diabetes. No one knows why some people with diabetes develop complications while others live with the condition for 50 years or more without developing complications. However, the latest research shows that good control of both blood glucose levels and blood pressure can greatly reduce the risk of complications arising, and many complications can be treated if they are detected soon enough, so it is important to be aware of the warning signs.

Eleanor

'I've been going to the eye clinic for about three years. I was told I would have to have my cataracts removed, but the operation had to be postponed, and when I went back they found there was bleeding at the back of my eye. That was a terrible blow because I'd always enjoyed reading. My great fear is that it will get worse and I'll be able to do less.

'I live in a shadowy world. My diabetes was diagnosed quite late, and I think my eyes were already affected before I realised.'

Why can diabetes lead to complications?

Over the years, diabetes can sometimes affect the large and small blood vessels of the body, causing damage to the tissue. Large blood vessel damage (sometimes called *macroangiopathy*) can affect anyone but is more common in people with diabetes. But small blood vessel damage (sometimes called *microangiopathy*) only affects people who have diabetes and some other rare conditions. This is more likely if the diabetes is not properly controlled.

Complications of large blood vessels

The arteries that carry the blood around the body can be damaged by diabetes. The most common form of large blood vessel disease is *atherosclerosis*, which means hardening of the arteries. It happens when fatty deposits of cholesterol build up on the inside of the arteries. Artherosclerosis is very common in Western societies – we probably all have some degree of it. But people with diabetes are particularly at risk.

Others at risk are people with high blood pressure, smokers and people who are overweight. People of Asian and Afro-Caribbean origin are also more at risk. If someone has diabetes they should try to minimise their other risk factors by watching what they eat, taking exercise and cutting out smoking.

When the arteries harden and get narrow, it means the organs and limbs served by them get less oxygen and can suffer damage. The way the different parts of the body are affected is discussed below ('Some common complications of diabetes').

Complications of small blood vessels

The fine blood vessels or capillaries, which bring oxygen right into the cells of the body, can become blocked or damaged in people with diabetes. The organs most at risk when small blood vessels are damaged are the kidneys and the eyes. Some people's nerves are also affected.

No one knows why some people with diabetes are more likely to develop complications affecting the eyes, nerves and kidneys, but high blood glucose level, high blood pressure, and how long someone has had diabetes are all risk factors. Family history also seems to play a part, so if someone in your family has had diabetes leading to eye or kidney complications it is particularly important to look out for warning signs.

Some common complications of diabetes

Heart disease

The heart works like a pump, pumping blood rich in oxygen around the body. To do this, the heart needs a good supply of blood itself, especially during exercise. When the blood supply to the heart is affected by damage to the blood vessels (see above), the heart will not get enough oxygen to function properly. The result is heart disease. Signs of heart disease include pain in the chest, extreme breathlessness and swollen ankles. However, if someone has any or all of these signs it does not mean they have heart disease – they can all be caused by many other factors. But it is wise to let the doctor know, so that the heart can be properly checked, and heart disease treated if necessary.

Hazel

Hazel's mother has angina and heart failure along with diabetes. Her father used to look after her, but at 85 it's getting too much for him.

'Lately Mum's started feeling very low. She doesn't want to get dressed in the morning. She can just make her way from the bedroom to the living room, and that's about it. I used to try and get her out of the house, but she's losing her confidence. She had a bad angina attack in the supermarket, and now she won't go out at all.'

Angina pectoris

The most common kind of heart disease is angina pectoris. This is severe pain in the chest brought on by exercise or stress, which goes away when the person rests. Angina pectoris can be successfully treated with a number of drugs.

Coronary thrombosis

This means that one of the main (coronary) arteries that brings blood to the heart is partially or completely blocked by a small clot (thrombus). The result is a heart attack (see below).

Myocardial infarction (heart attack)

This is what happens when the blood supply to the heart is partly or completely blocked by a small clot (see above) and an area of heart muscle dies. The usual signs are intense pain in the centre of the chest, sometimes reaching down the left arm, and sweating, pallor and breathlessness. If this happens it is important to call an ambulance at once.

Heart failure

This is when the valves of the heart are not working properly. The usual signs are breathlessness and/or swollen ankles. It does not mean the heart is suddenly going to stop working, but it does mean the person needs to see a doctor and get treatment.

Preventing heart disease

Heart disease is one of the main causes of death in the United Kingdom, and people with diabetes are especially vulnerable because of damage to their large and small blood vessels. But heart disease is also one of the most preventable diseases if people take the right steps soon enough. There are four key things everyone can do to prevent heart disease:

- Stop smoking.
- Eat a healthy diet.
- Take enough exercise.

■ Get to a reasonable weight and stay there.

There is more about this in Chapter 3.

High blood pressure (hypertension)

Someone is said to have high blood pressure when their heart has to work extra hard to force the blood through their arteries. This may be because the arteries are damaged or clogged with a fatty deposit called cholesterol. High blood pressure is common in the whole population, but people with diabetes tend to have higher blood pressure than most. Smoking, being overweight and stress can all contribute to high blood pressure, as can eating a high salt diet. There are no particular symptoms of high blood pressure, but if it is not treated it can lead to heart disease, kidney damage or stroke.

High blood pressure is treated with a range of drugs which are usually very effective. Someone with diabetes should have their blood pressure checked at least once a year.

Stroke

A stroke happens when the blood supply is cut off to part of the brain. This is usually caused by a clot in one of the arteries leading to the brain or by a burst blood vessel in the brain. A minor stroke, called a transient ischaemic attack, may not do much damage, but a more severe stroke may make the person partially paralysed on one side and affect their speech. With good and careful treatment and rehabilitation it is often possible to recover all or most of the movement and speech which have been lost.

Strokes are more likely to happen if someone's arteries are damaged through atherosclerosis (see p 69) and, once again, people with diabetes are more at risk. Controlling weight and blood pressure are particularly important in preventing strokes.

Foot problems and peripheral vascular disease

People with diabetes can easily get problems and infections in their feet that they are not aware of because their nerves have been damaged. That is why it is important to check the feet every day. There is more about foot problems and foot care in Chapter 7.

Eye problems

Retinopathy

Diabetes sometimes causes damage to the small blood vessels that bring blood to the retina. This is called *retinopathy*. (The retina is the network of nerve fibres at the back of the eye, which send visual messages to the brain). No one knows for sure why some people with diabetes get retinopathy while others do not. Heredity may play a part – diabetic retinopathy seems to run in families. But controlling blood glucose level and blood pressure levels and having a regular eye examination can help prevent damage to the eyesight. Unfortunately some people are not diagnosed with diabetes until there is already some damage, but even then, prompt laser treatment can often stop their eyesight getting worse.

Checking for retinopathy

People with diabetes should have their eyes checked when they are first diagnosed and then have regular eye examinations at least once a year. This is because there may be no symptoms of retinopathy until quite a lot of damage has already been done.

The eye examination for someone with diabetes is not the same as a regular eye test – it is concerned mainly with examining the retina at the back of the eye. First the pupils have to be dilated with special drops, then the ophthalmologist or optician shines a light through the pupil to examine the back of the eye for signs of damage. Sometimes a photograph is taken, so that there is a permanent record against which to track later changes and damage to the retina.

Treating retinopathy

If retinopathy is not treated it can lead to gradual loss of sight or eventually to blindness. However, if it is caught early enough, it can be very effectively treated. Laser beams are used to seal off the leaking or damaged blood vessels to the retina and prevent new abnormal blood vessels from growing. Most people who have had laser treatment are delighted with the result.

Ron

Ron is in his 70s, and has had diabetes since he was 43. In the last few years he has started having problems with his eyes.

'They told me I've got retinopathy. I've been for laser treatment three or four times. They give you a local anaesthetic, then they shine the laser beam in through your eye, and it seals off the blood vessels that are bleeding.

'But recently I had a bad haemorrhage at the back of my right eye. I was bending over doing something in the garden, and it went quite suddenly. They had to do an operation where they took out part of the jelly of the eye and replaced it with artificial jelly. That was very good – it restored my eyesight back to what it was before – but it only lasted for about seven months. Then something went wrong, and they said they couldn't do anything else. Now I'm getting a cataract in the same eye, but they don't want to take it out, because they say it won't make any difference. They're still giving me laser treatment in my left eye, and that isn't too bad. But it's a worry. I used to enjoy gardening, but now I'm a bit nervous about bending over like that in case I get another haemorrhage.'

Blurred vision

Blurred vision can be quite alarming because people sometimes think it's a sign that their eyesight is going. In fact it is usually caused by a change in the blood glucose and once the blood glucose level has been stabilised, the blurred vision will probably improve within a few weeks. High blood pressure can also cause blurred vision. Again, this should improve once the blood pressure is brought down. When someone starts taking insulin for the first time, this can also lead to blurred vision for a while.

Cataracts

A cataract is when the lens of the eye becomes hard and cloudy, making the vision foggy or blurred. Cataracts are quite common in older people, but they are up to five times more common in people with diabetes and tend to develop at an earlier age.

Cataracts can be treated by a simple operation to remove the lens, but this is usually only necessary when the vision is badly affected or if the cataract is getting in the way of laser treatment.

Eleanor

Eleanor has cataracts as well as retinopathy. 'They've been very good at the eye clinic. They are going to give me some more laser treatment, and after that I'll have a cataract operation on the other eye. Now I'm quite hopeful that I'll be able to see again.'

Glaucoma

Glaucoma is a rare condition caused by a build up of pressure at the front of the eye, which over time can lead to tunnel vision and blindness. It is more common in people with diabetes, and tends to run in families. Although the damage caused by glaucoma cannot be reversed, treatment can prevent the condition from getting worse.

For more *i*nformation

i *Diabetes and your eyes* and *Diabetes and visual impairment* available from the British Diabetic Association.

A note about getting new glasses

Diabetes often causes changes in eyesight, and when treatment begins the eyesight may change yet again. Too much glucose in the blood can cause blurred vision, while starting using insulin can change the refraction of the lens of the eye. It is worth waiting until a few weeks into treatment before having an eye test for new glasses, so that the eyes have had a chance to settle down.

Kidney damage

The kidneys filter the waste substances produced by the body through thousands of tiny tubules called *nephrons*, from where the waste passes down as urine into the bladder. Diabetes can damage the fine blood vessels that feed the nephrons, so they can no longer do their job. This is called *diabetic nephropathy*. One of the first signs of this is usually protein in the urine (*proteinuria*), which the doctor can detect with a simple dipstick test. If the kidney damage gets worse, the person may start feeling tired and breathless, and their ankles may start to swell.

If someone has nephropathy it is very important that they keep their blood pressure and blood glucose levels down. If there are signs of fluid retention, the doctor may prescribe diuretics. Eventually some people suffer kidney failure and need to be treated with dialysis, or they may be fortunate enough to be offered a kidney transplant.

Val

Val is in her 50s and has had diabetes since she was 18. Four years ago she started feeling very unwell.

'I started getting swelling in my ankles. Then one day my legs swelled up like balloons. The doctor didn't know what it was. He tried me on different medications, including tetracycline. I was living on Lucozade and little did I know that was making things worse, because Lucozade is very high in potassium. Then one day I collapsed and they rushed me into hospital, and they diagnosed kidney failure at once. I don't know why they hadn't realised what it was before.

'They put me straight onto haemodialysis, and that was my life for the next two years. It took 3-4 hours each time, and I had to go three times a week. At the end I would feel drained and exhausted. I felt really low. But then the consultant told me about CAPD (Continuous Ambulatory Peritoneal Dialysis) which I could do at home. It filters the fluids rather than the blood, so it is much less tiring. I have a bag of fluid, and I have to drain the old fluid out and let the new fluid drain in. It takes three quarters of an hour, and I have to do it four times a day, every day of the week. I've got it set up in the back bedroom, with a little TV. It's not nearly as tiring as the haemodialysis I had in hospital. And the beauty of it is, when we go away we can take it with us. We've got a little chalet down south and we can go down there when the weather's nice. And the CAPD comes with us in the car.'

Urinary tract and kidney infections

People with diabetes are also very prone to urinary tract infections, which can sometimes spread to the kidneys. The signs of urinary tract infection are a burning sensation on passing urine, and urine that is smelly and cloudy. If this happens, see the doctor straight-away, and antibiotics will be prescribed to prevent a kidney infection developing.

Nerve damage

Diabetes can damage the nerves that carry messages from the organs and limbs of the body to the brain. This is called neuropathy. For example if nerves in the hands or feet are damaged, the person may gradually lose their feeling of pain or heat or cold, or they may occasionally feel pain or a burning sensation for no apparent reason. If someone has damage to their nerves, particularly in their feet, they should be very watchful for any signs of broken skin or injuries, and seek medical advice at once, as they may have hurt themselves without being aware, and infection can very easily set in before they know it.

Hazel

'Mum can't feel her feet at all any more – she's lost the feeling about a quarter of the way down below her knees. And yet even though she can't feel anything, she still has a lot of pain. It's a burning pain she feels all the time. The doctor gives her tablets for the pain, but she can't take too many because they make her constipated.'

For more *i*nformation

ℹ *Diabetic neuropathy* produced by the British Diabetic Association.

Impotence

Sometimes in men, the nerves that send signals to the penis can be damaged, and the man will find it difficult to get or keep an erection. Impotence is quite common in men as they get older, but it is much more common in men with diabetes. It can be treated in a number of different ways, so it is important to talk to the doctor.

For more *i*nformation

ℹ *Impotence and diabetes* produced by the British Diabetic Association.

Damage to the autonomic nervous system

People with diabetes can also suffer damage to the autonomic nervous system. This is the part of the nervous system that we do not consciously control – it governs body functions such as sweating, sexual arousal, balance, and bladder and bowel control. All these can be affected by diabetes, though the symptoms are usually annoying rather than dangerous. The danger signals that warn someone they are about to have a 'hypo' can also be affected.

Note Reading about all these possible complications of diabetes can seem very depressing. But remember, not everyone gets all the complications, and some of them are quite rare. Most complications of diabetes are becoming much rarer, as better treatments are developed and the importance of maintaining a healthy blood glucose level is better understood.

Going into hospital

People have very different experiences of being in hospital. If the person you care for needs to go into hospital, whether or not their admission is to do with their diabetes, the staff should be informed that the person has diabetes so that they can offer appropriate care. The charge nurse should explain to you and the person you care for what is going to happen during their stay in hospital, and discuss how diabetes monitoring and control will fit into their overall treatment.

Keeping up the treatment/monitoring routine

You should let the hospital staff know the details of your relative's routine of meals, monitoring, and taking tablets and/or insulin. There may be some aspects of care, such as blood or urine monitoring or taking tablets or self-injecting, which he or she can carry on doing. However, insulin may need to be given as a drip directly into a vein, especially if the person you care for has to have an anaesthetic for an operation and cannot eat.

People who do not normally take insulin as part of their treatment are sometimes put on insulin temporarily while in hospital. This could happen if their illness or operation has temporarily upset their diabetes control, and it does not mean they will always have to be on insulin once they are out of hospital.

Emergency supplies

Patients who have diabetes will usually be allowed and encouraged to have their own emergency supply of snacks or drinks or glucose gel to hand in their locker in case they feel a 'hypo' coming on. Make sure the person you care for has what they need, and that the ward staff know it is there.

Keeping the diabetes team informed

Check that the specialist diabetes team at the hospital – the doctors, nurses, dietitian and chiropodist – know that your relative has been admitted so they can keep an eye on him or her, and take the opportunity for any additional treatment, care or monitoring.

Arrangements for discharge

Before the person you care for is allowed home from hospital, it is the hospital's responsibility to make sure that they will be able to cope once they get home. If necessary, the hospital social worker should liaise with you and with the council's social services department to make sure that someone will be there to look after them, and that any adaptations have been made to the home, especially if the person will be in a wheelchair.

If you are concerned about whether the person you care for will be able to manage at home, ask to speak to the social worker at the hospital, and prepare to be persistent if necessary. There are supposed to be clear procedures for discharging someone who needs continuing care from hospital, but each local authority and health authority has its own rules about discharge procedures.

Someone may be discharged from hospital once their medical condition has stabilised, even though they still need continuing nursing care. This has led to situations where people who thought they had a right to be cared for by the NHS were suddenly faced with huge bills for private care in a nursing home. If you are worried about this, contact Age Concern for advice.

For more *i*nformation

ⓘ Age Concern Factsheet 37 *Hospital discharge arrangements and NHS continuing health care services.*

ⓘ *Diabetes: What care to expect in hospital* and *Coping with diabetes when you are ill* leaflets available from the British Diabetic Association.

Audrey

Audrey had had diabetes for six years when she broke her hip while on holiday and had to be rushed to hospital. 'They put me on a drip for insulin while I had the operation. They gave me an epidural – they wouldn't give me a total anaesthetic. Then in the morning they brought me a needle and let me do my own injection. I was glad to be off the drip.

'But one thing that really upset me after I'd had the operation was that I wet the bed. And the nurse came and told me off. She made me feel like a naughty child. I said, "How can you talk to me like that? Do you realise how old I am? I'm away from home. I've had an operation. I've had an epidural, so I can't feel anything below the waist. I think it's most unkind." I told the staff nurse, and the other nurse came and apologised. But then I got an infection in the wound which caused me a lot of problems. I was so glad when they brought me home at last. They brought me in an ambulance and as I came over the Pennines the sun came out.'

People with diabetes are particularly vulnerable to infection, and, like Audrey, they should be prepared to complain if the treatment they get is not what it should be.

If you need to complain

Most people are satisfied with their treatment under the National Health Service, but if your relative has been badly treated you should consider making a complaint. No one likes to complain, but if you can point out what has gone wrong without being rude or aggressive, you can help make things much better for other people in future. It's best first to make your point informally to the person in charge. If you feel you haven't been listened to, ask about the complaints procedure. Every hospital and social services department has its own complaints procedure, and they should be able to give you a leaflet explaining how to take your complaint forward. If your complaint is serious, or you feel you are getting nowhere, the Community Health Council (known as the Health Council in Scotland) for that area will help you to make a formal complaint. They will be listed in the telephone directory, or the local NHS trust will have their number.

Protecting against infection and flu

People with diabetes may have particular trouble shaking infections off. This applies to common infections, as well as the rarer infections that can be picked up in hospital. Infections that seem quite trivial to most people can become serious for someone with diabetes, as they can rapidly put the blood glucose level up.

If the person you care for has even a quite common infection, such as flu or an upset stomach, you should keep an eye on them to make sure they do not develop symptoms of *hyperglycaemia* (see Chapter 8). Cuts, wounds and skin infections need to be treated with great care. If there is any sign of infection setting in, see a doctor or nurse straightaway. It is easier to prevent an infection developing than to clear it once it has taken a hold.

Another way to protect against infection is to make sure that the person you care for has a *flu jab* at the start of the winter. The practice nurse at the GP surgery will organise this. Ask the GP whether a vaccination against *pneumonia* would also be a good idea.

7 Foot care for someone with diabetes

People with diabetes are prone to have problems with their feet and legs. As a carer, one of the most important things you can do is keep an eye on the feet of the person you care for, and help them take care of their feet to prevent complications developing.

Hazel

'Mum was in her 80s when she started to have problems with her feet. She used to bang them a lot. We didn't realise it was because she was gradually losing all feeling in her feet. That was when her diabetes was diagnosed. Now they've put her on insulin she feels much better, but she still has pain in her feet. I help her look after her feet – I wash them every day and rub them with cream. I try and keep them soft and supple. The funny thing is, even though she can't feel anything in her feet, they still give her a lot of pain.'

Understanding problem feet

People with diabetes are more likely than most to develop foot problems – sometimes it is a problem in the feet or toes that leads to diabetes being diagnosed in the first place. Unfortunately foot problems are also one of the most common reasons for an older person with diabetes to be admitted to hospital.

Foot problems can happen because of poor circulation. If there is not enough blood circulating to the feet, injuries heal more slowly and it is harder to fight off an infection.

At the same time, people with diabetes sometimes suffer from neuropathy – damage to the fine nerves. Neuropathy can cause tingling or numbness in the feet, or the person may lose sensation in their feet altogether. So if they do cut or hurt their foot, or their shoes or slippers do not fit well, they may not realise there is anything wrong. They may carry on walking on the foot, leading to more damage and infection.

If a foot problem is allowed to develop untreated it can lead to pain, ulceration, gangrene, and even in extreme cases to amputation. So it is very important that someone with diabetes takes good care of their feet.

Everyday foot care

Keep feet dry and clean – check them daily

Keeping feet clean, dry and comfortable can help avoid damage and infection. Make sure the person you care for washes their feet gently in warm water and soap every day. Sometimes older people find it difficult to reach down to wash their feet, and this is something the carer can do for them. After washing, make sure all the soap is rinsed off and dry carefully, especially between the toes, taking care not to pull the toes apart too much. Use talcum powder very sparingly, or don't use it at all, as it can get clogged between the toes and encourage infection to develop. A gentle massage with an emollient cream such as E45 is a pleasant way to finish off the foot care routine. But do not apply cream between the toes as this area is usually moist enough.

Washing feet daily also means you are more likely to notice any problems (see 'Problems to look out for' below).

Take care of toenails

Toenails should not be so long that they rub or cut into the toes. But do not cut them too short, or dig down at the side of nails – this can lead to skin damage or ingrowing toenails. The best way to cut toenails is straight across to the shape of the toe, not in a curve going down at the sides. Any sharp edges should be gently filed away. Cutting toenails once every six to eight weeks is usually enough.

Older people often find it difficult to reach down and cut their toenails, especially if they also have arthritis. This is something the carer can help them with. It is best to cut toenails after a bath, when they are softer, and to use special toenail clippers. But if the nails are very thick or difficult to cut, or if there is neuropathy and loss of sensation in the toes or feet, it is better to ask the chiropodist rather than risk damaging the feet by doing it yourself. The GP or practice nurse will be able to tell you whether you should cut toenails yourself or go to a state registered chiropodist.

Protect your feet

Never walk barefoot – your feet need to be protected all the time.

Check shoes and socks before you put them on. Look out for bits of grit and stones, and places where the shoe is rough or could rub.

Make sure socks are the right size, and wear them inside out, so the seams don't rub or cut into the feet.

Don't wear slippers all day. They don't give feet enough support.

Avoid extreme hot or cold

Don't let someone's feet get too hot or too cold — make sure they wear warm shoes or boots and thick socks or long johns if they go out in cold weather. People with diabetes often suffer with cold feet. But warming up chilly feet on a heater or in front of the fire or putting them straight into warm water can lead to burns and skin damage. Put warm dry socks on instead, and let the feet warm up gradually. Be careful that bath water is not too hot. Always test the temperature with the elbow, not with the hand or foot.

Problems to look out for

Someone with diabetes needs to check their feet every day to look out for tell-tale signs that something is going wrong. If they find it hard to bend down to see their feet, it is something the carer can do for them.

■ Look out for changes in colour in the feet – especially the toes. If any of the toes seem to be turning red, blue, brown or black see the doctor or go to the clinic at once.

■ Look out for sore spots, cracks, corns, blisters, callouses or veruccas (these look like a brown or black spot in the centre of an area of hard skin). Flaking skin and sore cracks under the toes may be a sign of athlete's foot. Weeping from the toenail may be a sign of infection under the nail.

■ Check for any swellings in the feet or legs.

■ Be aware of any strange or unpleasant smell – this can be a sign of infection.

■ Note sores or broken skin on the leg or foot – these can develop into an ulcer.

If you notice any of these changes, don't leave it until the next appointment – seek help urgently from the diabetes clinic or your GP. It is surprising how fast an infection can develop in the feet once it gets a hold.

Don't attempt to deal with corns and callouses yourself. You could easily damage the skin and cause an infection. People with diabetes can see a state registered chiropodist free of charge (look for the letters SRCh after the chiropodist's name).

Some older people hate to make a fuss over things which seem trivial, or they may say that it can't be anything serious because it doesn't hurt – but that in itself can be a sign that something is wrong. It's better to get a professional opinion than to risk having to have toes or feet amputated.

Val

Val has had diabetes since her teens, and knew she had poor circulation when problems started to develop. 'I had an ulcer down on my leg above the ankle that just wouldn't clear up. It was weeping and sore. Then one of my toes went black. The doctor said there was just not enough blood getting down to my ankle to let it heal up. It ended with me having to have the leg amputated. Then a year or so later I got the same problem in the other leg, and that had to be amputated as well. It was a dreadful blow.'

Choosing shoes

Shoes should be comfy and snug-fitting. Shoes that are too tight can cause pressure sores, callouses and damage to skin and joints. Shoes which are too loose can rub or let the feet slide about, causing extra damage. So it's important to get the fit just right. A warm or fleecy lining can provide extra cushioning, and can help to keep the feet warm – important when circulation is a problem. Shoes or boots with laces or a buckle are best as they stay on the foot securely and are less likely to rub. Velcro fastenings can be useful for someone whose fingers are arthritic or neuropathic, but velcro can loosen and stretch as it wears, so check that it is still giving good support. Choose a style of shoe which is the shape of the foot. Some women's styles, especially those that are cut low on the foot such as court shoes, can cut into the foot or rub on the heel or squeeze the toes.

Monica

Monica is a diabetes specialist nurse specialising in foot care. She says: 'You can't depend on a person with neuropathy to tell you whether a shoe fits or not, because they can't feel it. They need to have their feet measured. People with neuropathy are often more comfortable in shoes which are a bit too small, so asking them how the shoes feel is no use at all.'

When you go out shopping for shoes with the person you care for, make sure they try on plenty of pairs before they buy. Ask a trained shoe-fitter to measure the person's feet for length and width – this should be done while they are standing up, not sitting down. There should be a bit of room at the end of the big toe when they stand up in the shoe. Make sure they practice walking in them as well as sitting and standing. Shoes that crease across the top when they walk may be too narrow.

If the person has bunions, corns or callouses, or if you have trouble getting shoes to fit, ask a state registered chiropodist about special pads and insoles, or about getting special shoes on the National Health Service.

You should be able to find shoes which are comfortable, well fitting and well made in an ordinary High Street store, but the chiropodist or the clinic will also be able to tell you of specialist shops which stock shoes for problem feet. Never buy shoes by mail order.

Hazel

'My Mum was having so much trouble finding shoes to fit, and the doctor at the hospital was worried about the nerve endings in her feet. In the end they gave her a special pair on the NHS. In fact she got two pairs, a beige pair for the summer and a navy pair for the winter. They aren't the most glamorous – the style is like a trainer – but they're extra width, and very comfortable.'

For more *i*nformation

- *i* Call the British Diabetic Association Careline on 0171-636 6112.
- *i* *Taking care of your feet* published by the British Diabetic Association.

8 Coping with emergencies

When you are caring for someone with diabetes, you need to know what to do if something goes seriously wrong with their blood glucose level. This chapter describes what happens when someone has hypoglycaemia (low blood glucose, commonly called a 'hypo'), and what happens when they have hyperglycaemia (high blood glucose). However well someone controls their diabetes, there will be times when their blood glucose level goes too high or too low, and you need to know what to do.

Clive

'The first time, it was terrible. They hadn't warned me it can make you wet yourself or mess yourself. If you fall over in the street, people assume you're drunk, and they ignore you. But now I know if I need to eat. I feel very low – it's like a clock that's beginning to wind down. I get speckles in front of my eyes, and I begin to feel cold and clammy. When that happens, I just have a bite of a Mars bar.'

Hypoglycaemia

When someone is taking insulin or certain tablets to control their diabetes, their blood glucose level can sometimes dip too low. This is called hypoglycaemia, or 'having a hypo' or 'going hypo'. Having a 'hypo' is quite common, and most people with diabetes will have recognised and treated it themselves successfully. Going 'hypo' is not usually dangerous in itself, but it can have dangerous effects, for example if the person hurts themselves while falling. It can also be extremely unpleasant.

Although 'hypo' symptoms, and the blood glucose level at which they arise, vary from person to person, they fall into certain common patterns and are often constant for each person. Most people start to become hypoglycaemic when their blood glucose level drops below 4 mmol/l, but some people can feel a 'hypo' coming on at a higher level, depending on their diabetes control.

Getting exactly the right balance between food, exercise and insulin or tablets is not easy. The better someone is at keeping their blood glucose level down, the more at risk they may be that it will go too far down, and they will go 'hypo'. However, most people have warning signs that a 'hypo' is coming on, and if they recognise the signs and take some sugary food or drink straight away they will be all right.

Some people worry about having a 'hypo' at night. If the person wakes up feeling shivery or sweating or feels very hungry they may be going 'hypo' during the night. If this happens regularly, suggest a snack before going to bed. If you can, check the blood glucose level during the night. Reassure the person that having a 'hypo' at night is not dangerous – it will gradually wear off as the insulin level goes down.

People who are controlling their diabetes with diet alone, or with diet and certain tablets, are not likely to have a 'hypo'. If you are not sure about the type of tablets the person you care for is taking, ask the doctor or nurse.

What can cause hypoglycaemia

Someone with diabetes risks going 'hypo' if he or she has:

- taken too much insulin;
- taken too many sulphonylurea tablets, or taken them too close

together (see Chapter 4 for more information about taking tablets to control diabetes);
- skipped a meal or snack, or had a meal later than usual;
- taken a meal or snack which did not have enough carbohydrate;
- taken more exercise than usual, or some other strenuous activity;
- drunk alcohol on an empty stomach.

Signs of hypoglycaemia

The signs listed below are all signs that someone's blood glucose level may have slipped too low. The person may experience one or more of the following:

- tingling around the mouth;
- trembling;
- irregular heartbeat;
- blurred vision;
- headache;
- turning very pale;
- feeling faint or weak;
- feeling hungry;
- feeling irritable or grumpy;
- confusion;
- slurred speech;
- strange behaviour;
- unsteadiness;
- poor co-ordination and concentration.

As the body tries to correct the low blood glucose, it releases a hormone called *adrenaline*. This in turn can cause:

- sweating;
- rapid heartbeat;
- feelings of anxiety or panic.

Audrey

'It's a dreadful sensation. I get very dizzy. Sometimes I feel nauseated. My eyesight goes funny, my legs go – then that's it. I'm out on the floor. Very often I'm sick. It leaves you feeling lifeless. I'm always afraid that I'll have one when I'm out.'

If the symptoms go on, and the person does not take preventative action, then they may become unconscious or even have a fit. In a small number of people on insulin, hypoglcaemia can occasionally cause more dangerous and alarming symptoms such as temporary paralysis, tongue biting, or fitting. This is obviously very frightening, though it is comforting to know that the person will recover completely

Val

'You can't describe it. You start sweating. Your mind is muffled. I find my mind is racing through things – then I go out. When I come round I'm absolutely soaking and shivering with cold, and I feel so sick. Then I feel hungry – I feel I could eat a horse.'

Usually people with diabetes are good at recognising the signs of a 'hypo' and take preventative steps themselves. But sometimes they get confused or irritable and refuse to take anything. It's sometimes the carer or other friends or family members who recognise the warning signs and insist that the person takes some sugar or glucose.

What to do

Give the person the simplest short-acting carbohydrate available. This is the instant cure for all the symptoms above. This could be in the form of:

- a glass of fruit juice;
- glucose tablets or Hypostop gel;
- a sweet sugary drink (NOT a 'diet' or 'light' drink);
- jam or honey;
- sweets or chocolate (these may take a little longer to act).

Glucose tablets or gel are fast-acting, and you can buy them from the chemist. Make sure there are some around the house, and that the person you care for carries some with them whenever they are out.

When someone has experienced a 'hypo' once or twice, they will soon learn to recognise their individual symptoms, and they will know whether their 'hypo' is mild or more severe.

Mild hypo

If the person is feeling irritable or confused, or has just started to experience mild 'hypo' symptoms described on page 91:

Immediately take:	Followed by one or two of the following:
3 or more glucose tablets or	a sandwich
5 sweets, eg barley sugar, or	fruit
glass of fruit juice or	biscuits and milk
glass of Lucozade or coke	bowl of cereal and milk
(not diet drinks)	

Moderate hypo

When someone has a moderate or severe 'hypo' they will probably need help.

You can get glucose gel from the chemist. It comes in many brand names. Keep a supply in the house just in case.

Immediately take:	Followed by one or two of the following:
4 or more teaspoons of honey or	as above
4 or more teaspoons of treacle or	
a sugar gel (eg Hypostop)	

If the person is unconscious or has a fit:

- Call an ambulance immediately – tell the emergency service that there is a person with diabetes who is unconscious.
- Place them in the recovery position (on their side with their head tilted back so that the tongue doesn't block the throat).
- Don't try to make them eat or drink anything.
- Don't try to get them up.
- Stay with them until help arrives.

To bring the person round quickly, you can give them a Glucagon injection. This is a natural hormone that releases glucose from the liver. Ask the doctor or specialist nurse about using Glucagon, and if necessary keep a supply in the house. (If you give Glucagon, and the person comes round and makes a good recovery, there is no need to call an ambulance.) Once the person is conscious, they should take carbohydrates by mouth.

Don't panic. Remember, most people recover quite naturally from a 'hypo' even if you don't do anything. Their body will slowly respond by naturally increasing blood glucose levels, and the person will eventually become conscious again as the effect of the insulin or tablets wears off.

After a 'hypo'

The person may feel weak and weepy, or they may feel very tired and low.

Audrey

'Coming round from a 'hypo' is the worst. You feel very emotional. You feel you've let yourself down. It makes you aware that there is something wrong with you.'

Talk it through with the person and try to work out why they had a 'hypo'. Did they miss a meal or a snack, or have it too late? Did they take their tablets at the wrong time? Did they tire themselves out doing shopping, or get out of breath running for the bus? Understanding why it happened can help prevent it happening next time.

If the person seems to be having a lot of 'hypos' tell the doctor or specialist nurse – their medication may need to be adjusted.

For the carer, too, watching someone have a hypo can be very distressing.

Keith

'The first time I saw Val having a hypo I didn't know what was happening, and I was terrified. She blacked out and fell on the floor, and all her limbs were jumping about like an epileptic fit. I panicked. I didn't know what to do so I rushed into the kitchen for the sugar jar, but I couldn't find it. So I called the doctor.

'Now I'm better prepared. We have Hypostop (a glucose gel) in the house, or I can give her a Glucagon injection. When she comes round I give her little sips of water so she doesn't get dehydrated if she's been sick.

'I think it's important for the carers to see someone going into a hypo, to prepare them for what to expect.

'I let the children see Val having a hypo. Although it's upsetting, it's better for them to realise that it's something that can happen, so they know what to do.'

Hyperglycaemia

When someone has too much glucose in their blood this is called hyperglycaemia. Usually once diabetes has been diagnosed and is being treated, the blood glucose level will not go too high (for most people, a blood glucose level of between 4 and 10 mmol/l is all right). But occasionally something can happen, usually when the person has another illness or infection, that can send the blood glucose level soaring. When this happens, it means someone is not getting enough insulin for their needs, and hyperglycaemia is the result.

If someone becomes severely insulin-deficient their body fat begins to break down into *ketones*. These make the blood acid, and if the person is not treated they may become very drowsy, confused and ill and eventually slip into a coma. Ketones are a sign that diabetes is seriously out of control. Ketones are likely if someone is vomiting, and can very quickly make them feel even worse. You can get special testing sticks called Ketostix to check the urine for ketones, and the doctor can prescribe these for someone with a tendency to hyperglycaemia (more usual in type 1 diabetes). If a ketone test is positive, contact the GP or diabetes team immediately. Sometimes you can tell someone is becoming *ketotic* because their breath has a sweetish pear-drops smell, but not everyone is aware of this smell, so do not assume everything is all right because you don't notice it.

Once diabetes is being treated, hyperglycaemia is much less common than hypoglycaemia, but it can be much more serious. It usually happens when someone has another illness or infection. Illness and infection almost always increase blood glucose level, so someone may need more insulin or tablets than usual. A common error people make is to stop taking insulin if they are feeling ill. The combination of infection and reduced insulin intake can soon put someone's blood glucose level up.

If the person you care for is taking insulin, keep a close watch on them if they have another illness, even something quite common such as flu or an upset stomach. Get treatment for any skin wounds or infections that do not heal up straightaway. **Above all, make sure they never miss a dose of insulin or tablets**.

What can cause hyperglycaemia

Someone may become hyperglycaemic if:

■ they have been taking tablets for diabetes but have not been able to keep them down due to vomiting;
■ they have not taken insulin which was prescribed for them;
■ they have another illness or infection which has put their blood glucose level up.

Signs of hyperglycaemia

Hyperglycaemia generally comes on more slowly than hypoglycaemia. It usually takes at least a day before you notice any signs. The person you care for may be becoming hyperglycaemic if they:

■ feel constantly thirsty;
■ need to pass urine a lot.

If either of these happens, contact the doctor or specialist nurse as soon as possible for advice.

If the person

■ feels sick or starts to vomit;
■ feels drowsy;
■ breathes rapidly and shallowly;
■ has flushed, dry skin;
■ seems to be slipping into a coma;
■ has breath that smells of pear drops.

THIS IS AN EMERGENCY. DIAL 999 FOR AN AMBULANCE OR RUSH THE PERSON TO HOSPITAL

What to do about hyperglycaemia

Hyperglycaemia is very serious. If someone has the symptoms listed above, they should be rushed to hospital.

If the person has mild signs of hyperglycaemia regularly, such as thirst and passing a lot of urine, get them to see their doctor urgently, as it could mean that they need to change their medication.

Clive

'When Audrey's diabetes was first diagnosed, her blood glucose was out of control. It was awful. I could hear her moving about upstairs, and then there was a crash, and she'd fallen down. One day I came back from work and found she'd blacked out. I rang the ambulance, and the two paramedics couldn't bring her round. They rushed her to hospital and put her on an insulin drip.

'People get the symptoms, but they don't know what they mean. They drink a lot and pee a lot – they don't realise it's a classic sign of high blood glucose.'

For more *i*nformation

i   Call the British Diabetic Association Careline on 0171-636 6112.

9 Looking at the long term

One of the hardest things about being a carer is having to make long-term decisions without knowing what the future will bring. This chapter looks at the way your situation could change over time, and how this could affect decisions about caring. It tells you what help you could get from the council to carry on caring at home, and looks at other possibilities if caring at home becomes too difficult.

Annie

'When I look back, I realise that he was starting with Alzheimer's at the same time as he got diabetes. He kept on forgetting things. But I wasn't aware of it at the time. Then one day we went out for a walk, and suddenly he went rushing off. I tried to follow him, but I got out of breath and had to sit down. Then he came back and said, "I want to go home. Give me the key." He rushed off again. He was behaving so strangely, I knew something was wrong. I took him to see the doctor, who asked him a lot of questions. He could answer some, but not others. The doctor took me on one side and said, "I think he's got a bit of dementia." The doctor told me my husband's Alzheimer's was not related to the diabetes. But it made looking after him much harder.'

Thinking about the future

As you and the person you care for both grow older, the way you care may need to change and develop too. Three things that are almost certain to change over time are:

- the health of the person you care for;
- your own health and stamina;
- your relationship with the person you care for.

Will the person need a lot more care in the near future? Will you perhaps need care yourself? Will you start to resent the amount of time and effort you put into caring? Or will you start to become more dependent on the person you care for? Thinking about these issues can help you start planning for the future.

The health of the person you care for

Diabetes affects people differently, so no one can predict how the health of the person you care for will bear up. So long as the diabetes is well controlled and there are no complications, most people can manage well. However, if someone starts to develop severe complications that affect their eyesight or mobility, they will become more dependent on those around them.

Diabetes and other health problems

All of us are liable to develop health problems as we grow older. Older people with diabetes can develop other health problems that are unrelated to their diabetes, such as arthritis or Alzheimer's disease.

Try to talk to the GP or hospital consultant about the long-term health outlook of the person you care for. They cannot make exact predictions and they are bound by rules to keep the confidence of their patients. But they may be able to describe how someone's condition changes with diabetes and how it can interact with other health problems.

Your own health and stamina

Caring for someone can be a stressful and demanding job, and many studies have shown that carers are more likely to suffer ill health than other people.

Annie

Annie found that her own heart condition made it much harder to keep up with her husband's wanderings. 'He would go rushing off, and I would hurry after him as best I could. But I just couldn't keep up. Once I collapsed on my neighbours' doorstep. I was so breathless I could hardly get the words out, but when they realised what had happened they went after him in the car and brought him back. Another time he went out wearing his carpet slippers in the pouring rain, and he fell down near the church. I managed to get him back and get him in dry clothes. But I knew I couldn't cope any more. So I started to lock the doors to stop him rushing off. After that, I always lived behind locked doors. It was heartbreaking.'

You may need help if:

- you need to lift or turn the person, and they are too heavy for you;
- the person cannot be left alone for more than an hour or so;
- the person needs personal care which you don't feel able to give;
- the person needs care from a doctor or nurse;
- you find caring for the person very stressful;
- you have to look after the person day and night.

Under the Carers' Act (1995), if someone is assessed as needing care, the carer is also entitled to an assessment of his or her needs. There is more about assessment on page 103.

Your relationship with the person you care for

The relationship between a carer and the person they care for is a very intense one. Often there is a range of different emotions all mixed together – love, anger, guilt, gratitude, resentment, commitment, irritation, to name but a few. As time passes, the balance in the relationship may change. For example children end up looking after their parents. A husband or wife who was once very dominating can end up being the weak and helpless one. This can bring up new emotions. Sometimes tenderness or gratitude, sometimes anger and resentment come to the surface.

People often feel very guilty about their negative emotions. But if you are caring for someone, it is best to accept that you are only human. You must look for a way of caring that fits in with your life, and does not require you to be a saint.

Marie

When Marie's husband was diagnosed with diabetes she found it hard to forgive the way he had behaved in the past.

'He's not been the best of husbands. He used to drink a lot, and was physically abusive. Now I'm left holding the baby. I don't resent looking after him – what I resent is the 40 wasted years of our marriage.'

Getting help with care

Whether you are caring for someone who lives with you, or for someone who lives elsewhere but needs you to pop in regularly, you may be able to get help. The NHS and Community Care Act (1990) encourages ways of caring for people in their own home if it means they would otherwise have to live in a care home.

The social services department of the local authority is responsible for what they call 'social care' – that means practical care with getting up, getting washed and dressed, using the toilet, cooking and eating – in fact everything you would normally do for yourself. However, you may be expected to contribute to the cost of the care.

The voluntary sector and charities such as Age Concern may also be able to help with social care. Your area Health Authority Trust (Health Board in Scotland) is responsible for any medical or nursing help you need. This is free (unless you choose to go privately).

How social services can help

If managing at home has become a daily struggle, you can ask the local social services department to carry out an *assessment* to see what help they can offer.

Usually, someone will come to your house and go through a series of questions to find out what kind of help the person needs. They will want to know how well they can manage to look after themselves, and also what medical care they need. They will look at where the person lives, who else lives there, and what help and support there is from other family members. Finally, they will also ask questions about the person's finances, to find out how much they should pay towards the cost.

When they have made their assessment, they should come up with a *care package* of services they can arrange to help the person manage better. If you are caring for someone who is being assessed, and you feel you need extra help, don't forget to ask for an assessment of your own needs.

Help you may be able to get through social services

- Assessment of your relative's needs.
- Support at home, including:
  - someone to help the person you care for get up and dressed in the morning;
  - someone to help them get to bed at night;
  - someone to help with personal care and bathing;
  - someone dropping in regularly to check they are all right;
  - someone to help with domestic tasks;
  - someone to make sure your relative takes their medication regularly.
- Meals on wheels; some local authorities provide this service themselves, but many now buy it in from other providers.

■ Regular care at a day centre; some day centres also offer meals, baths, hairdressing, chiropody, education classes and social activities.

■ Occupational therapist to advise about aids and alterations at home.

■ Respite care. This could be:
  – someone coming to sit in while you go out for a few hours;
  – someone sleeping in overnight occasionally to give you a good night's sleep;
  – somewhere for the person being cared for to stay for a week or two while the carer has a break.

■ Help finding residential care or nursing home care if necessary.

Note Most local authorities offer some of these services, but there may be a long waiting list and there may be a charge.

How voluntary and charitable groups can help

Voluntary and charitable groups such as Age Concern and the British Diabetic Association can offer support to carers. Many national groups have local branches (see 'Useful Addresses' pp 123–132). In addition some church or community groups can help in their local area.

To find out what is available in your area, ask at the diabetic clinic or ask your social worker if you have one. The Citizens Advice Bureau, the local community centre, local library or church can also be good sources of information.

National organisations may help with:

■ information about a particular illness or disability;
■ your rights regarding benefits and services;
■ advice about money and legal matters;
■ making a complaint;
■ campaigning for a better deal.

Local groups or local branches of national groups can help with:

- luncheon and social clubs;
- sitting service – someone to sit in while you go out for an hour or two;
- care at home;
- meals on wheels;
- community transport – volunteers take people shopping, or to a day centre or hospital;
- befriending schemes and 'good neighbour' schemes (someone regularly visits a lonely person at home);
- support groups for carers.

Note Although voluntary and charitable groups are non-profit making, most of them have to make a charge for the services they provide, to cover their costs and volunteers' expenses.

Getting help privately

Not everyone can afford private help. But it can cost less than you think to buy in extra help at home or to create more flexibility for the carer.

Help you may be able to buy privately

- Paid carers or help coming to your home – contact by word of mouth or by advertising or through an agency.
- Help with shopping – a local shop may deliver; some supermarkets provide transport for shoppers. The milkman may deliver other items such as dairy products, bread, potatoes, tea, etc.
- Laundry – there are agencies which collect and deliver laundry, or your local launderette may do a service wash if someone can take and collect it (but they may not accept very soiled laundry).
- Taxis – some taxi firms offer reduced rates for pensioners.
- Occasional take-out meals delivered to the door (the occasional pizza with a low-fat topping and served with salad can be a healthy choice for people with diabetes!).
- Nursing care through a nursing agency.

■ Physiotherapy or speech therapy through an agency or through the hospital.

■ Use of facilities in private residential or nursing homes, eg walk-in showers or special bathing facilities, hydrotherapy pool, etc. Many homes are happy to let non-residents use their facilities for a fee.

■ Care in a residential or nursing home (either long-term or respite or day care).

Note Do not feel you have to pay for a service if it is essential – the local authority should provide it. If some of the services listed above would make all the difference to enabling someone to live independently at home, ask for it when their needs are assessed.

For more *i*nformation

ⓘ Age Concern Factsheet 6 *Finding help at home.*

Getting your home adapted

Most older or disabled people want to carry on living in their own home. The thought of pulling up roots and going to a different place can be very worrying and upsetting, especially if it means losing their independence and going into a care home.

Alterations such as a stair-lift, wider doors for wheelchair access, a downstairs lavatory or a walk-in shower can make all the difference to helping an older or disabled person keep their independence.

Occupational therapist assessment

An occupational therapist (OT) is trained to look at how people with disabilities can manage everyday tasks such as getting about, washing, using the toilet, cooking, preparing drinks, eating, etc, and to suggest ways these could be made easier. OTs can be based either in a hospital or in the social services department of your local authority. If you are considering having any alterations to make life easier for a disabled person, try to get an OT's advice first. And if you want to apply for a *disabled facilities grant* (see below) then you will have to get an OT to say that the alterations are essential.

Unfortunately OTs are in short supply in many areas and there can be quite a wait for this service.

Keith and Val

When Val had both her legs amputated in hospital, she was desperate to get home as soon as she could. But the hospital would not let her home until grab rails and a ramp were installed at their bungalow. Said Keith, 'It was so frustrating – Val wanted to be home, and I wanted her home. She was perfectly well and she didn't want to be lying in a hospital bed, just waiting. So in the end I did it myself. I put a ramp in at the front door, and I put grab rails in the bathroom and toilet. But not everyone can do that – so they have to stay in hospital for weeks. No wonder there's a shortage of beds.'

Keith and Val also had a long wait for an electric hoist to be installed in the bathroom. 'We got it through the NHS and we had to wait for months,' said Val. 'I couldn't have a bath, so I had to make do with a wash down. That was really getting to me, and making me feel depressed. But now I've got the electric hoist which I can work myself, and I'm much more independent.'

Grants from the council

Alterations can be expensive, but you may be able to get a grant from the local authority towards the cost. Most grants are means-tested, so they will depend on the home owner's income and savings. There are two kinds of grants: **mandatory grants** are the grants the council has to pay if the work qualifies and a person's income and savings are low. With **discretionary grants** it is up to the council to decide whether to give them or not.

Renovation grants are discretionary grants, paid for essential repairs to make a property structurally safe and habitable, and to provide essential services such as lighting, heating and ventilation, cooking facilities, clean drinking water, an indoor toilet, a bath or shower with hot and cold water and drainage.

Disabled facilities grants can provide facilities for a disabled person. They may be mandatory if they are for specified purposes.

Home repair assistance grants are discretionary grants, available for smaller repairs and alterations, such as providing insulation or draught proofing. You can also get grants for alterations to enable a person over 60 to move into a carer's home, such as installing a downstairs toilet. These grants are normally only available to people on benefit. If the work costs more than the amount of the grant, you will have to make up the difference yourself. These grants are not available in Scotland.

Note Don't start alteration work before getting the go ahead from the council, or you will automatically be disqualified from receiving a grant.

For more _i_nformation

- _i_ Contact your local authority's housing or environmental health department for advice about grants. If the person you care for is a tenant, they should talk to their landlord about applying.

- _i_ **Care and Repair** and **Staying Put** are agencies that have been set up specially to advise older people and people with disabilities about repairing and adapting their homes. To find out whether there is a project near you, look in the telephone directory, or ask your local housing department, or contact Care and Repair Ltd (address on p 125).

- _i_ Age Concern Factsheet 13 _Older home owners: financial help with repairs and adaptations_.

- _i_ _An Owner's Guide: Your Home in Retirement_, published by Age Concern Books (now out of print, but may be available in libraries).

- _i_ Carers National Association Factsheet 1 _Gadgets and Equipment to Aid Daily Living_ (address on p 125).

Choices about where to live

There may come a time when the person you care for finds they can no longer manage where they are. It may be that they can no longer manage stairs, or their home is unsuitable for a wheelchair. Maybe it is no longer safe for them to live alone. Having their home altered or adapted (see above) can be the ideal solution for some people, but it does not suit everybody.

This section looks at some of the other choices open to you and the person you care for.

Sheltered housing

For older people who do not need full-time care, but who would like someone nearby to keep an eye on them, sheltered housing could be the perfect answer. These developments of flats or bungalows are specially adapted for the needs of older or disabled people, with a warden either on-site or dropping in regularly. Some are linked to an alarm system. If the person you care for is considering a sheltered housing scheme, check exactly what help the warden gives, as this can vary greatly. The warden does not usually help with care, but will alert someone in an emergency. Some people ask for sheltered housing near where they live at present, while others choose to move near to their family.

There are two main problems with sheltered housing. Firstly, it is very popular, so it tends to be in short supply. Secondly, it is mostly available for rent, and the rents are quite high, so it may only be suitable for people on a low income if they are entitled to housing benefit. People who own their own homes may find the rent is more than they can afford unless they sell their home and spend or invest the capital.

Some schemes are council-run, some are private, and many are run by voluntary organisations. Some private sheltered housing developments have flats or bungalows for sale.

For more *i*nformation

i The Housing Department at your local authority has information about all sheltered housing schemes in your area, not just council-run schemes.

i Age Concern Factsheet 2 *Retirement housing for sale*.

i Age Concern Factsheet 8 *Rented accommodation for older people*.

i Help the Aged Information Sheet No 2 *Sheltered Housing*.

i *Housing Options for Older People* by David Bookbinder, published by Age Concern Books (now out of print, but may be available in libraries).

Abbeyfield homes

The Abbeyfield Society is a charitable trust that divides large houses into bedsits for older people. There is a resident house-keeper who provides two cooked meals a day, and some other bills are also covered. The cost may be a little higher than in ordinary sheltered housing, but it is ideal for someone who wants to combine independence with some companionship.

The Abbeyfield houses have up to about ten bedsits suitable for fairly active and independent people aged over 75, who do not need personal or nursing care, but who can no longer manage to run their own household. Some Abbeyfield houses now provide extra care for more dependent people.

For more *i*nformation

i Contact the Abbeyfield Society – look in your local telephone directory under Abbeyfield Homes Society, or see p 123.

Living with the carer

If you are caring for an elderly relative or friend, you may be considering inviting them to come and live with you, or buying a property where you can live together. This can be a good arrangement for some people, but it is a very big step and needs a great deal of thought if it is to be successful.

If you really like the company of the person you care for, and know that you won't get irritated with each other, then it could work well. But if your main reason is a sense of duty or obligation, then you will probably find the arrangement begins to break down, however fond you are of the person. You could try living together on a temporary basis first to see how you get on, maybe for a month's 'holiday'.

Sometimes an arrangement where people live close by but have their own separate living space works better for everybody.

Eleanor

Eleanor is going to live near one of her daughters. 'I feel so lucky. They have adapted a flat for me above the office where she works, so there will always be someone around during the day. I'm not worried about living by myself – I've done that for years – but I like to know there's someone close by, especially as I get older.'

For more *i*nformation

ⓘ *Caring at Home* by Nancy Kohner, published by National Extension College.

ⓘ *Who Cares Now? Caring for an older person* by Nancy Kohner and Penny Mares, published by BBC Education.

Residential or nursing home care

Many older people say that they dread 'going into a home'. They don't like the thought of being cared for by 'strangers' and they worry about loss of privacy and independence. The carer, too, may see care in a home as 'putting someone away', and feel they have failed in their duty. However, for some people, a residential or nursing home is the best or the only option. If the person you care for needs residential care, it is much better to concentrate on

111

finding a good home that meets all their needs than to blame yourself or feel guilty about it.

Your local social services department can give you a list of homes in your area, and advise about which ones might be suitable. But you and the person you care for will want to satisfy yourselves that the home is a good one, where residents are well cared for, and their dignity respected.

Choosing a home

There are plenty of books and guides that can advise you about choosing a home. Some are listed below. Before you set out and visit a lot of homes, there are some basic questions you can ask over the phone, which can save you a lot of footwork:

- Is the home registered with the local authority?
- Does the home provide residential or nursing care? (see p 111)
- Would they accept the person you care for? (Not all homes can take someone who is very disabled, and some do not take people with Alzheimer's disease.)
- Can they cater for a person with diabetes? Do they have any experience of looking after people with diabetes?
- How many residents are there, and how many staff? Who is there at night?
- Who owns the home, and who is responsible for its day-to-day running?
- Is the location right? Is it convenient for you to visit?
- What are the fees? Are there any extras?

Asking these questions can help you narrow down the number of homes you visit. If a home sounds promising, you could ask them to send you a brochure.

It's best to visit three or four homes before you decide. Involve the person you care for, even if they cannot visit all the homes with you. Never assume that their tastes and priorities are the same as yours – you may dream of a room with a view, while they like to see people going by the window. You may like a bright modern décor while they like an old-fashioned look. You may like friendly and informal staff – they may feel a more formal tone is more dignified. Make sure the home fits their ideas as well as yours.

Things to look out for in a home

■ Do you like the person in charge? Do you feel at ease with her or him?

■ What are the other staff like? How long have they been there? How do they behave towards the residents?

■ Does the home look and smell clean and fresh?

■ What are the other residents doing? Are they busy and active, or are they sitting passively in chairs around the walls of a day room?

■ What are the other residents like? Would the person you care for fit in?

■ How many of the residents have dementia? (It can be upsetting for someone who is physically unwell but mentally alert to be living in a home where the majority of residents have dementia.)

■ Is there a homely atmosphere? Are there flowers, pets, indoor plants? Is the décor pleasant and cheerful?

■ Is the room you have been offered large enough and attractively decorated? Can residents bring their own possessions?

Some people recommend visiting at a meal time, to give you a feel for the atmosphere in the home, and the relations between staff and residents. Remember, paying the staff a decent wage costs more than a new coat of paint and pretty curtains. But cheerful friendly staff who have a long-term commitment to their job and to the residents make all the difference to the residents' experience.

Paying for residential or nursing home care

Your local social services department should first assess whether the person needs to be cared for in a home and whether they need residential or nursing home care. Residential homes provide personal care such as washing, dressing, using the toilet and help with meals and eating (all the things someone would do for themselves if they were able). Nursing homes provide full nursing care from a qualified nurse.

Care in a residential or nursing home can be very expensive. Fees range from about £200 per week in a residential home to £600 or more in a nursing home, depending on where you live and the amount and kind of care you need. However, many people can get some help from the Department of Social Security (DSS) and the local authority towards the cost.

The social services will look at someone's income and their capital and savings (assets). If they have assets of less than £16,000 and their weekly income is less than the fees of the home, the local authority will make up the difference between the person's total weekly income and the cost of the home. However, if someone has assets over £16,000 they will have to pay the full cost of the fees until their assets drop down to this amount. And any savings between £10,000 and £16,000 will be taken into account in assessing their income.

Married couples are assessed separately. If savings or assets are held in joint names, the local authority will assume that half belongs to each spouse.

If someone owns their own house or flat, its value could be counted as part of their assets unless their spouse is still living there, or another relative who is aged over 60 or disabled.

Caring in a care home

When the person you care for goes into a home, it is not the end of your caring role – you just start to care in a different way. Sometimes it is better to show your love by letting go but staying involved, and working with the home to make sure your relative gets the best possible care.

Annie

Annie could cope with her husband's diabetes, but when he developed Alzheimer's as well she found looking after him increasingly difficult. 'My daughters and the social worker persuaded me to let him go into respite care during the day, and then to stay for a week in every month. I didn't want to let him go, but it got that bad. He used to wee and do his business on the floor. He didn't mean to, but he couldn't help it. Sometimes he would get a bit violent with me from time to time, but I didn't tell anybody, because I didn't want them to take him away. The social worker said it might be better if he went into residential care, but I always said no. I said, "I married him for better or worse."

'Then one night he started to wee in his chair, and I told him to go to the toilet. And he started to shout at me, saying "Who do you think you are?" Then he picked up a cushion and started to hammer me. I was terrified, but he's much stronger than me, and he wouldn't let me go. I managed to crawl out of the window. I rang my daughter, but by the time she got here he'd gone to the respite home. Then they rang me from the home and said it would be better if he stayed a couple of weeks. Then at the end of the fortnight they said it would be better if he stayed permanently. I was heartbroken. I used to stand by the window waiting for him to come home.

'They know he has diabetes at the home, and they keep up his diet. Sometimes we help feed him, and we've noticed they bring him extra fresh fruit, instead of a pudding. They watch out for any signs. They do their best to work with us, and we work with them.

'I go to see him every week. Some days he recognises us, some days he doesn't. To me it's like a living bereavement. I've lost him, yet I've still got to care for him. We've had 56 years of happy marriage. He's looked after us all these years – now it's our turn to look after him.'

For more *i*nformation

i *Finding and paying for residential and nursing home care* by Marina Lewycka, published Age Concern Books (details on p 134).

i Age Concern Factsheet 10 *Local authority charging procedures for residential and nursing home care.*

i Age Concern Factsheet 11 *Financial support for people in residential and nursing home accommodation prior to 1 April 1993.*

i Age Concern Factsheet 25 *Income Support and the Social Fund.*

i Age Concern Factsheet 29 *Finding residential and nursing home accommodation.*

i **Counsel and Care** is a voluntary organisation that gives advice and information about voluntary and private residential homes (address on p 127).

i Counsel and Care Factsheet No 19 *Paying the fees of a registered private or voluntary home for people who entered the home on/after 1st April 1993.*

i Counsel and Care Factsheet No 17 *What to look for in a private or voluntary registered home.*

i **Elderly Accommodation Counsel** provides computerised advice about finding and paying for housing for older people (address on p 128).

i **Relatives Association** is a voluntary organisation for relatives who have a family member in a care home. It advises about staying involved and working with the home to improve the quality of care (address on p 129).

Glossary

Here are some words and phrases you may come across at the doctor's or in hospital.

A

Acetone A chemical substance (one of the ketones) with a sweet smell that develops in the body when diabetes is poorly controlled and fat and protein stores are being used for energy. It is passed in the urine where it can be detected by testing, and it can also be smelt on the breath.

Acidosis A build-up of acids, usually ketones, in the blood.

Adrenalin Hormone which is released in response to stress. Causes an increase in blood glucose levels.

Albumin A protein which, if found in the urine, may indicate either infection or early signs of kidney damage.

Alcohol-free drinks Contain very little alcohol. This type of beverage may also be high in sugar.

Alpha cells Produce glucagon found in Islets of Langerhans.

Arteriosclerosis Hardening and narrowing of the arteries which occurs with advancing years in those with or without diabetes.

Artificial, or intense, sweeteners Products which provide an intense level of sweetness and are calorie-free. They provide a suitable replacement for sugar. Examples are saccharin, aspartame, acesulfame potassium.

B

Beta cells Another name for the insulin producing cells.

Blood glucose Level of glucose (sugar) in the blood.

C

Calorie (kcal) A standard measurement of heat or energy used to assess the energy value of food.

Carbohydrate (CHO) A class of foods that is an important source of energy to the body. It is mainly represented by sugars and starches.

Cataract Cloudiness and opacity of the lens of the eye which affects sight.

Chiropody Treatment of foot problems.

Cholesterol A type of fat found in blood, related to cardiovascular disease.

Coma A state of unconsciousness. In diabetes this can result from severe hypoglycaemia or severe ketoacidosis.

D

DCCT Stands for Diabetes Control and Complication Trial. An American study which was set up to compare the effects of two different types of insulin regime on the development and progression of diabetic complications.

Dehydration Refers to being depleted of water. It occurs when blood glucose is high for long periods as in ketoacidosis.

Dextrose A simple sugar.

Diabetes mellitus The full name for diabetes.

Dietary fibre A complex mixture of different substances found in plants, eg fruit, vegetables and wholegrain foods.

F

Fat atrophy Disappearance of fat from under the skin, at the site of insulin injection. More common with older insulins.

Fat hypertrophy Fatty swelling occurring when insulin is being injected repeatedly into one area.

Fructosamine A blood test which reflects the average blood glucose levels over the previous two to three weeks.

G

Gangrene Death of tissue due to poor blood supply.

Glucagon A hormone produced by the pancreas. It raises the blood glucose level and can be given by injection to correct hypoglycaemia.

Glucose A simple sugar.

Glycogen The form in which carbohydrate is stored in the liver.

Glycosuria The presence of sugar in the urine.

H

Haemoglobin Alc (glycosylated haemoglobin) A test used to assess long-term diabetic control over the previous two months. Often known as HbAlc.

Honeymoon period The short time after diagnosis when the dose of insulin is reduced due to the partial recovery of insulin secretion from the pancreas.

Hormone The name given to a chemical substance released by a gland into the bloodstream. Hormones are responsible for controlling such functions as metabolism, growth, sex development, blood glucose levels, etc.

Hyperglycaemia A high blood glucose level (more than 10 mmol/l).

Hypoglycaemia or 'hypo' A low blood glucose level (less than 4 mmol/l).

I

IDDM Stands for Insulin Dependent Diabetes Mellitus. Now more commonly known as type 1 diabetes.

Insulin A hormone produced by the beta cells in the Islets of Langerhans in the pancreas. It enables glucose in the blood to get into the cells and be used for energy or stored.

Insulin reaction Another term for hypoglycaemic reaction.

Intestine The gut or bowel between the stomach and the anus.

Intravenous glucose Glucose delivered directly into a vein.

Ischaemia Lack of blood supply to body tissue or organs. Can occur if blood vessels are constricted or blocked.

Islets of Langerhans See Insulin, Pancreas.

K

Ketoacidosis or ketosis A state of over-production of ketones in the body which causes a build-up of acids in the blood. May lead to 'diabetic coma'.

Ketones Ketones are produced when fats are broken down in the body. If a lot of fat is broken down, as in poorly controlled diabetes, the ketones accumulate in the blood, pass into the urine and can be smelt on the breath.

Ketonuria The presence of ketones in the urine.

L

LDSAG Stands for Local Diabetes Services Advisory Group.

Lactose The simple sugar found in milk.

Lipids Group of fats in bloodstream – see Cholesterol and Triglycerides.

Lipohypertrophy Fatty swelling usually caused by repeated injections of insulin into the same site, also known as fat hypertrophy.

Low alcohol beverages Have a reduced alcohol content, but are not alcohol free. These drinks can be high in sugar.

M

Mmol/l Millimols per litre, a measure of the concentration of a substance – usually the amount of glucose in the blood.

Monitoring Regular testing of blood or urine to check control of diabetes.

Monounsaturated fats Have beneficial effects with respect to heart disease. This type of fat is found mainly in olive, nut and rapeseed oil.

N

NIDDM Stands for Non-insulin Dependent Diabetes Mellitus. Now more commonly known as type 2 diabetes.

Nephropathy The medical term for kidney damage which may occur as a result of long-term diabetes.

Neuropathy A disorder of the nerves which affects their signalling function; this can be a complication of diabetes.

O

Ophthalmologist An eye specialist.

Oral hypoglycaemics Tablets prescribed for people with non-insulin dependent diabetes.

P

Pancreas A long organ lying across the back of the abdomen. Part of it secretes digestive juices into the intestine, but its Islets of Langerhans, pinpoint-sized collections of cells scattered throughout it, secrete insulin and glucagon.

Photocoagulation Treatment of retinopathy by laser light.

Polydipsia Excessive thirst and desire to drink; a symptom of untreated diabetes.

Polyunsaturated fats Thought to be beneficial with regard to heart disease. These are found in sunflower, corn and soya oil and margarine labelled high in polyunsaturates.

Polyuria Passing of large quantities of urine. In diabetes this is due to excess glucose from the bloodstream being filtered by the kidneys. A symptom of untreated diabetes.

Post-prandial After a meal.

Protein A major food component important in body growth and repair.

Pulses Edible seeds of certain plants of the legume family, eg beans, peas and lentils.

R

Renal threshold The level of glucose in the blood at which glucose 'spills' into the urine.

Retina The light-receptive layer at the back of the eye. It is an extension of the optic nerve in the eye.

Retinopathy Damage to the retina; a complication of long-standing diabetes.

S

Saturated fats Have been linked with the development of high cholesterol levels and heart disease. These fats are found in meat and meat products, dairy products, cakes, biscuits and pastries.

Sucrose Common form of table sugar. Sucrose can be included, in small amounts, as part of a healthy diet.

T

Thrush A fungal infection of skin, mouth or vagina; can be a symptom of undiagnosed, or poorly controlled diabetes.

Triglyceride A form of fats used to carry or store fats in the body.

U

Unit Refers to a quantity chosen as a standard basic measurement of insulin.

V

Vitamins Compounds found naturally in small quantities in foods. They are required for normal growth and maintenance of life, although they do not themselves provide energy or nourishment.

Glossary reproduced by kind permission of the British Diabetic Association from their magazine *Balance for Beginners*.

Useful addresses

Abbeyfield Society
53 Victoria Street
St Albans
Hertfordshire AR1 3UW
Tel: 01727 857536
Housing association specialising in bedsits for older people in shared houses with meals provided.

Alzheimer's Disease Society
Gordon House
10 Greencoat Place
London SW1P 1PH
Tel: 0171-306 0606
Information, support and advice about caring for someone with Alzheimer's disease.

Alzheimer's Scotland -- Action on Dementia
22 Drumsheugh Gardens
Edinburgh EH3 7RN
Tel: 0131-220 6155
24-hour helpline: 0800 317 817
Information and support for people with dementia and their family and carers in Scotland. Supports a network of carers' groups.

Arthritis Care
18 Stephenson Way
London NW1 2HD
Tel: 0171-916 1500
Advice about living with arthritis, loan of equipment, holiday centres. Local branches in many areas.

Arthritis Research Campaign
Copeman House, St Mary's Court
St Mary's Gate
Chesterfield
Derbyshire S41 7TD
Tel: 01246 558033
Medical research charity dedicated to finding not only the cause of arthritis, but also the cure.

British Association of Cancer United Patients (BACUP)
3 Bath Place
Rivington Street
London EC2A 3JR
Tel: 0171-696 9003
Support and information for cancer sufferers and their families. Freephone advice line for people outside London: 0800 181 199.

British Diabetic Association
10 Queen Anne Street
London W1M 0BD
Tel: 0171-323 1531
Careline: 0171-636 6112
Internet at: www.diabetes.org.uk
Provide help and support to people diagnosed with diabetes, their families and those who care for them.

British Diabetic Association Distribution Department
PO Box 1
Portishead
Bristol BS20 8DJ
Tel: 0800 585 088
Publications on all aspects of diabetes, and recipe books for people with diabetes.

British Heart Foundation
14 Fitzhardinge Street
London W1H 4DH
Tel: 0171-935 0185
Information about all aspects of heart disease.

British Lung Foundation
78 Hatton Garden
London EC1N 8JR
Tel: 0171-831 5831
Information about all aspects of lung disease.

British Red Cross
9 Grosvenor Crescent
London SW1X 7EJ
Tel: 0171-235 5454
Can loan home aids for disabled people. Local branches.

CancerLink
11–21 Northdown Street
London N1 9BN
Tel: 0171-833 2818
Freephone information: 0800 132 905
Asian freephone: 0800 590 415
Information and advice about all aspects of cancer.

Care and Repair
Castle House
Kirtley Drive
Nottingham NG7 1LD
Tel: 0115-979 9091
Advice about home repairs and improvements.

Carers National Association
20–25 Glasshouse Yard
London EC1A 4JS
Tel: 0171-490 8818 (1–4pm weekdays)
Information and advice if you are caring for someone. Can put you in touch with other carers and carers' groups in your area.

Chest, Heart and Stroke Association
See Stroke Association, British Heart Foundation and British Lung Foundation.

Chest, Heart and Stroke Scotland
65 North Castle Street
Edinburgh EH2 3LT
Tel: 0131-225 6963
Information about all aspects of heart disease, lung disease and stroke for people living in Scotland.

Northern Ireland Chest, Heart and Stroke Association
21 Dublin Road
Belfast BT2 7FJ
Tel: 01232 320184
Information about all aspects of heart disease, lung disease and stroke for people living in Northern Ireland.

Citizens Advice Bureau
Listed in local telephone directories, or in the *Yellow Pages* under 'Counselling and advice'. Other local advice centres may also be listed.
For advice on legal, financial and consumer matters. A good place to turn to if you don't know where to go for help or advice on any subject.

Community Health Council
See the local telephone directory for your area (sometimes listed under 'Health Authority/Board'). Called Health Councils in Scotland.
For enquiries or complaints about any aspect of the NHS in your area.

Continence Foundation
The Basement
2 Doughty Street
London WC1N 2PH
Tel: 0171-404 6875
Advice and information about whom to contact with incontinence problems.

Counsel and Care
Lower Ground Floor
Twyman House
16 Bonny Street
London NW1 9PG
Tel: 0171-485 1566 (10am–4pm)
Advice for elderly people and their families; can sometimes give grants to help people remain at home, or return to their home.

Court of Protection
Public Trust Office
Protection Division
Stewart House
24 Kingsway
London WC2B 6JX
Tel: 0171-664 7300
If you need to take over the affairs of someone who is mentally incapable (in England and Wales).

Crossroads Care
10 Regent Place
Rugby
Warwickshire CV21 2PN
Tel: 01788 573653
For a care attendant to come and look after your relative at home.

Dial UK (Disablement Information and Advice Lines)
Park Lodge
St Catherine's Hospital
Tickhill Road
Balby
Doncaster DN4 8QN
Tel: 01302 310123
Information and advice for people with disabilities. Can put you in touch with local contacts.

Disability Law Service
Room 241
2nd Floor
49–51 Bedford Row
London WC1R 4LR
Tel: 0171-831 8031
Free legal advice for disabled people and their families.

Disability Scotland
Princes House
5 Shandwick Place
Edinburgh EH2 4RG
Tel: 0131-229 8632
Information for disabled people living in Scotland.

Disabled Living Centres Council
Winchester House
11 Cranmer Road
London SW9 6EJ
Tel: 0171-820 0567
Can tell you the address of your nearest disabled living centre, where you can see and try out aids and equipment.

Disabled Living Foundation
380–384 Harrow Road
London W9 2HU
Tel: 0171-289 6111
Information about aids to help you cope with a disability.

Elderly Accommodation Council
46A Chiswick High Road
London W4 1SZ
Tel: 0181-995 8320
Helpline: 0181-742 1182
Computerised information about all forms of accommodation for older people and advice on top-up funding.

Health Services Authority
See your local telephone directory.
The body responsible for GPs and primary health care.

Holiday Care Service

2nd Floor, Imperial Buildings
Victoria Road
Horley
Surrey RH6 7PZ
Tel: 01293 771500 (admin)
Information helpline: 01293 774535
Free information and advice about holidays for elderly or disabled people and their carers.

Incontinence Information Helpline

Tel: 0191-213 0050
Information and advice about managing incontinence, and how to contact your nearest continence adviser.

Local Government Ombudsman

21 Queen Anne's Gate
London SW1H 9BU
Tel: 0171-915 3210
If you want to make a complaint about the local authority.

Parkinson's Disease Society

22 Upper Woburn Place
London WC1H 0RA
Tel: 0171-383 3513
Support and information for relatives and carers of someone with Parkinson's disease.

Relatives Association

5 Tavistock Place
London WC1H 9SS
Tel: 0171-916 6055
Advice, information and support for relatives of people in a residential or nursing home. Produces leaflets and offers a listening ear and opportunities to join or form local groups.

Royal Association for Disability and Rehabilitation (RADAR)
12 City Forum
250 City Road
London EC1V 8AF
Tel: 0171-250 3222
Information about aids and mobility, holidays, sport and leisure for disabled people.

Royal National Institute for Deaf People (RNID)
19–23 Featherstone Street
London EC1Y 8SL
Tel: 0171-296 8000
Minicom: 0171-296 8001
Information and advice about all aspects of hearing loss; information about hearing aids.

Standing Conference of Ethnic Minority Senior Citizens
5 Westminister Bridge Road
London SE1 7XW
Tel: 0171-928 7861
Information, support and advice for older people from ethnic minorities and their families.

Stroke Association
123–127 Whitecross Street
London EC1Y 8JJ
Tel: 0171-490 7999
Information and advice if you are caring for someone who has had a stroke.

United Kingdom Home Care Association (UKHCA)
42B Banstead Road
Carshalton Beeches
Surrey SM5 3NW
Tel: 0181-288 1551
For information about organisations providing home care in your area.

About the British Diabetic Association

The British Diabetic Association is the leading national diabetes charity. Our network of over 180,000 members, six regional offices, 450 branches and our friends allow us to provide help and support to the 1.4 million people currently diagnosed with diabetes, their families and those who care for them.

With the money we raise we:

- offer confidential help and support on all aspects of diabetes through our dedicated Careline;
- organise educational holidays and clubs for children of all ages and their families;
- invest over £4.5 million each year in research into the causes, effects, treatments and cure of diabetes;
- work to protect the rights and interests of people with diabetes in the UK, dealing with issues such as discrimination and healthcare provision;
- produce a wide range of publications covering every aspect of diabetes care and control;
- offer a comprehensive range of insurance and financial products created for people with diabetes, at a fair and affordable price, through BDA Services.

Become a member of the British Diabetic Association

At the heart of the British Diabetic Association are the members, who make all we do possible. Your membership helps fund our research, fight our campaigns and provide our services.

By joining, you will receive *Balance*, our bi-monthly magazine. You will have the support of the leading national diabetes charity and can contact our Careline on 0171-636 6112 (see p 124 for address) for free and confidential advice.

About Age Concern

Caring for someone with diabetes is one of a wide range of publications produced by Age Concern England, the National Council on Ageing. Age Concern cares about all older people and believes later life should be fulfilling and enjoyable. For too many this is impossible. As the leading charitable movement in the UK concerned with ageing and older people, Age Concern finds effective ways to change that situation.

Where possible, we enable older people to solve problems themselves, providing as much or as little support as they need. Our network of 1,400 local groups, supported by 250,000 volunteers, provides community-based services such as lunch clubs, day centres and home visiting.

Nationally, we take a lead role in campaigning, parliamentary work, policy analysis, research, specialist information and advice provision, and publishing. Innovative programmes promote healthier lifestyles and provide older people with opportunities to give the experience of a lifetime back to their communities.

Age Concern is dependent on donations, covenants and legacies.

Age Concern England
1268 London Road
London SW16 4ER
Tel: 0181-765 7200
Fax: 0181-765 7211

Age Concern Scotland
113 Rose Street
Edinburgh EH2 3DT
Tel: 0131-220 3345
Fax: 0131-220 2779

Age Concern Cymru
4th Floor
1 Cathedral Road
Cardiff CF1 9SD
Tel: 01222 371566
Fax: 01222 399562

Age Concern Northern Ireland
3 Lower Crescent
Belfast BT7 1NR
Tel: 01232 245729
Fax: 01232 235497

Other books in this series

Caring for someone with alcohol problems
Mike Ward
When drinking becomes a problem, the consequences for the carer can be physically and emotionally exhausting. This book will help anyone who lives with or cares for a problem drinker, with particular emphasis on caring for an older problem drinker.
£6.99   0–86242–227–2

Caring for someone at a distance
Julie Spencer-Cingöz
With people now living longer, sooner or later, we are likely to find ourselves looking after a loved one or a friend — often at a distance. This book will help you to identify the needs and priorities that have to be addressed, offering guidance on the key decisions to be made, minimising risks, what to look for when you visit, how to get the most out of your visits, dealing with your relative's finances and keeping in touch.
£6.99   0-86242-228-0

Caring for someone who has had a stroke
Philip Coyne and Penny Mares
Although 100,000 people in Britain will have a stroke this year, many people are still confused about what stroke actually means. This book is designed to help carers understand stroke and its immediate aftermath. It contains extensive information on hospital discharge, providing care, rehabilitation, and adjustment to life at home.
£6.99   0-86242-264-7

Caring for someone who has dementia
Jane Brotchie
Caring for someone with dementia can be physically and emotionally exhausting, and it is often difficult to think about what can be

done to make the situation easier. This book shows how to cope and seek further help as well as containing detailed information on the illness itself and what to expect in the future.

£6.99   0-86242-259-0

Finding and paying for residential and nursing home care
Marina Lewycka

Acknowledging that an older person needs residential care often represents a major crisis for family and friends. Feelings of guilt and betrayal invariably compound the difficulties faced in identifying a suitable care home and sorting out the financial arrangements. This book provides a practical step-by-step guide to the decisions which have to be made and the help which is available.

£6.99   0-86242-261-2

The Carer's Handbook: What to do and who to turn to
Marina Lewycka

At some point in their lives millions of people find themselves suddenly responsible for organising the care of an older person with a health crisis. All too often such carers have no idea what services are available or who can be approached for support. This book is designed to act as a first point of reference in just such an emergency, signposting readers on to many more detailed, local sources of advice.

£6.99   0-86242-262-0

Caring for someone who is dying
Penny Mares

Confronting the knowledge that a loved one is going to die soon is always a moment of crisis. And the pain of the news can be compounded by the need to take responsibility for the care and support given in the last months and weeks. This book attempts to help readers cope with their emotions, identify the needs which the situation creates and make the practical arrangements necessary to ensure that the passage through the period is as smooth as possible.

£6.99   0-86242-260-4

Publications from Age Concern Books

Money matters

Your Rights: A guide to money benefits for older people
Sally West
A highly acclaimed annual guide to the State benefits available to older people. Contains information on Income Support, Housing Benefit and retirement pensions, among other matters, and provides advice on how to claim.
For further information, please telephone 0181-765 7200

Managing Other People's Money (2nd edition)
Penny Letts
Foreword by the Master of the Court of Protection
The management of money and property is usually a personal and private matter. However, there may come a time when someone else has to take over on either a temporary or a permanent basis. This book looks at the circumstances in which such a need could arise and provides a step-by-step guide to the arrangements that have to be made.
£9.99   0-86242-250-7

Ethnic Elders' Benefits Handbook
Sue Ward
Written in clear and concise English, this book aims to help anyone from an ethnic minority understand how the Social Security benefits system works, what their rights are and how they can claim a benefit to which they may be entitled. It includes explanations of the legal issues covering immigration and citizenship.
£9.99   0-86242-229-9

Health and care

The Community Care Handbook: The reformed system explained (2nd edition)
Barbara Meredith
The delivery of care in the community has changed dramatically as a result of recent legislation, and continues to evolve. Written by one of the country's foremost experts, this book explains in practical terms the background to the reforms, what they are, how they operate and whom they affect.
£13.99   0-86242-171-3

Know your Medicines (3rd edition)
Pat Blair
This popular guide covers, in clear language, many of the common questions that older people – and those who care for them – may have about the medicines they use and how these may affect them.
£7.99   0-86242-226-4

If you would like to order any of these titles, please write to the address below, enclosing a cheque or money order for the appropriate amount made payable to Age Concern England. Credit card orders may be made on 0181-765 7200.

Mail Order Unit
Age Concern England
1268 London Road
London SW16 4ER

Information Line

Age Concern produces over 40 comprehensive factsheets designed to answer many of the questions older people – or those advising them – may have, on topics such as:

■ finding and paying for residential and nursing home care
■ money benefits
■ finding help at home
■ legal affairs
■ making a Will
■ help with heating
■ raising income from your home
■ transfer of assets

Age Concern offers a factsheet subscription service that presents all the factsheets in a folder, together with regular updates throughout the year. The first year's subscription currently costs £50; an annual renewal thereafter is £25. Single copies, up to a maximum of five, are available free on receipt of an sae.

To order your FREE factsheet list, phone 0800 00 99 66 (a free call) or write to:

Age Concern
FREEPOST (SWB 30375)
Ashburton
Devon TQ13 7ZZ

Index